GINSENG

How to Find, Grow, and Use
America's Forest Gold

Kim Derek Pritts

STACKPOLE
BOOKS

Published by
STACKPOLE BOOKS
5067 Ritter Road
Mechanicsburg, PA 17055

Printed in the United States of America

10 9 8 7 6 5 4 3 2 1

First edition

Cover design by Kathleen D. Peters

Library of Congress Cataloging-in-Publication Data

Pritts, Kim D. (Kim Derek), 1953–
  Ginseng : how to find, grow, and use America's forest gold / Kim Derek Pritts. — 1st ed.
    p.   cm.
  ISBN 0-8117-2477-8 (pb)
  1. American ginseng. 2. Ginseng. I. Title.
IN PROCESS
633.8'83687—dc20   95-7210
                                                              CIP

GINSENG

Kim Derek Pratt

In memory of Clifford N. Pritts
and his keen eye for good weeds

Contents

Preface

American ginseng is one of this country's best-kept secrets. Ginseng has been traditionally known as an Asian herb, so many people are surprised to learn that it is actually a native American. In fact, nearly all the world's supply of wild ginseng is located in the United States. And ginseng cultivation has become a reclusive multimillion dollar business in North America.

For me, ginseng has been a lifelong hobby. I started hunting ginseng before I knew how to spell it and fell in love with the shy, retiring plant immediately. After thirty years of digging and studying ginseng, I still get excited at the first glimpse of a gold-tinged ginseng leaf on a crisp September morning.

This book would not be complete if I did not take the opportunity to thank Paul Hsu, president of Hsu's Ginseng Enterprises, for his invaluable help in evaluating the commercial cultivation of American ginseng. During an extended visit to his Wausau, Wisconsin, ginseng farm, I found myself quite impressed with his delightful family, his business, and his insight into the ginseng trade.

Additional recognition is in order for the men and women of the U.S. Fish and Wildlife Service and the World Wildlife Fund for their assistance in compiling federal information. Last, but certainly not least, I want to tip my hat to the diggers, growers, and dealers across the United States who took the time to share good tales about ginseng with me.

In the pages that follow, you will find information on American ginseng and its various methods of cultivation. The neophyte ginseng enthusiast would do well to look closely at the investment potential of woodsgrown and wild-simulated ginseng. Total ginseng acreage under artificial shade is increasing, so that market may become saturated in the future. Woodland-cultivated ginseng that closely resembles our native wild ginseng is likely to show steady improvement in the face of dwindling natural supplies and increasing demand by the Oriental consumer. This is the market of the future for U.S.–origin ginseng. So take a look at the twenty-first century's exciting prospects for America's forest gold!

Introduction

A root of which the Chinese have long been extravagantly fond, has of late, I find, been recommended in this place [London]; and merits the greater consideration, as it is one of the products of our own colonies in North America. The name of this drug is ginseng. Some considerable parcels of the root have been sent to China, and disposed of to great advantage.

The Gentleman's Magazine,
London, May 1753

The earth's history has changed dramatically since that article appeared in England nearly 250 years ago, but one thing has remained constant over the centuries—the world's hunger for ginseng. American growers today produce nearly 2 million pounds a year of the wrinkled, gnarled root. Canadian growers add another 1.5 million pounds each year. And the Oriental countries produce ginseng in tonnage that dwarfs the North American production. A full 95 percent of this worldwide crop is consumed in the Asian marketplace. Yet Far East buyers eagerly demand even more—at prices that have reached $65 per pound for cultivated American roots and $300 per pound for wild American ginseng.

The question in most Western minds is, why?

Ginseng is the most revered medicinal plant in the world. From its first recorded use in China five thousand years ago, to the biblical mention of *pannag* (interpreted as *ginseng* by some scholars) in Ezekiel, to Daniel Boone's ill-fated adventures, to the Russian cosmonaut program, to the health consciousness of modern America, ginseng has spanned the ages as a constant in a world of change.

The claims are legendary. Ginseng has historically been touted as an agent to make old men young, an aphrodisiac, a tonic, and a panacea, or all-healing medicine. Chinese roots that resembled the human shape were, until as recently as thirty years ago, bestowed with mystical reverence. Humanlike roots with "legs" of equal length were judged to be most desirable, or male. Roots with unequal lower limbs were considered female.

Even the gathering of the man-root was steeped in mysticism during the early Chinese dynasties. Altars of tree limbs were often assembled near wild ginseng plants, and prayers were recited before the roots were unearthed.

In North America, the aromatic tubers were used by many Native American nations, including the Cherokee, Iroquois Six

Nations (Mohawk, Oneida, Onondaga, Cayuga, Seneca, Tuscarora), Delaware, Menominee, Potawatomi, Fox, Penobscot, Creek, Chippewa, Pawnee, and Sioux. This is not surprising, since Native Americans were true herbalists with an intimate knowledge of nature's many healing plants. Ginseng utilization, however, varied widely among individual tribes. To the Creek, a freshly chewed ginseng root was considered a potent wound dressing, while a concoction of ginseng root with ginger was used to counteract a fever. Ginseng tea was considered a cure for croup. There are even references to Creek use of ginseng as a ghostbuster—the root was employed to frighten away spirits. The Penobscot used ginseng as a fertility drug, and the Fox and Cherokee used it to treat female ailments. Both the Fox and Delaware prescribed ginseng for sexual problems and used it as a love charm. Members of several nations, including the Chippewa, Menominee, Potawatomi, and Fox, took ginseng as a tonic to enhance mental alertness. This "mental booster" aspect was particularly favored by the Menominee. The Potawatomi used ginseng as an eyewash and to treat earaches. A number of Indian tribes used ginseng for stomach disorders.

Although utilized in varying degrees by the different Indian nations, ginseng medicinal applications often mirrored those of the Chinese half a world away. Interestingly, there are some claims that, until export of American ginseng began in the eighteenth century, most Native American use of ginseng was limited to treatments for stomach disorders, eye inflammations, earaches, and bleeding wounds. The Asian-style employment of ginseng as a fertility drug, mental booster, and panacea may well have been assimilated into tribal customs after contact with Eastern traders who paid the Indians to dig ginseng. More recently, attention has turned to ginseng as a restorative agent and immune-system enhancer in the United States. And with alternative medicine increasing in popularity in America, the market for high quality ginseng is bound to grow.

Orientals are the major users of all varieties of ginseng worldwide. The Asian consumer has shown a preference for wild ginseng roots, or those that most closely resemble the wild roots. This, then, is the market to which cultivators must also cater. Of additional interest is the Asian distinction between the varieties of ginseng. The ginseng aficionados of the Far East view American and Asian ginseng as two related but distinctly different medicinal herbs.

The traditional Western attitude has been that ginseng is ginseng. The Chinese, however, have espoused for centuries that American and Asian ginseng roots have separate and distinctive genetic profiles. Recent scientific studies now validate the Chinese belief that, even though taxonomically similar, the two ginsengs are quite different chemically. Therefore, each variety has a unique niche in Chinese traditional medicine. American ginseng is viewed as yin, or cool and calming; Asian ginseng is seen as yang, or stimulating and warming. Our concern is with the outlook for American ginseng. If we are to invest in the future of ginseng, what lies ahead?

Just as the markets for sweet corn and field corn are vastly different, so too are the markets for various grades of ginseng. Chinese vendors recognize an incredible 141 grades of wild ginseng and 40 to 50 grades of cultivated ginseng. These grades span the range from priceless imperial Chinese ginseng to the lowly Japanese Tong Yong Sam. American ginseng falls somewhere in between. Roots are ranked by shape, texture, color, and weight. Measured medicinal properties have no bearing upon the grading or the ultimate value of ginseng roots.

The demand for American ginseng has fluctuated over the centuries, often influenced more by New World blunders than by any significant upheaval in world trade. First discovered in 1716 in Canada, American ginseng brought French-Canadian traders the equivalent of $5 per pound by 1752—a veritable fortune at the time. Greed, however, soon overshadowed good business sense, and immature roots scorched by improper drying were sent to China with no consideration for the consumer. The backlash against these inferior roots soured the Chinese merchants on Canadian-origin ginseng. The Canadian ginseng trade with China fell from $100,000 in the mid 1750s to a mere $6,500 by 1759. Then another more serious problem arose. The early Canadians found that their frenzied digging had nearly driven ginseng to extinction within their borders. It took scores of years for the market to recover. The old Canadian proverb *"C'est tombe comme le ginseng"* ("It went down like ginseng") gives stark testimony to the folly of avarice in the ginseng trade.

Some two hundred years later, Canada is back in the ginseng business in a big way. Government-subsidized ginseng farms are increasing their production every few years, offering more and more competition for the U.S. ginseng market. Nearly all Canadian ginseng is cultivated under artificial shade, however, and is in direct competition with only our own field-cultivated ginseng. U.S.–origin woodsgrown, wild-simulated, and wild American ginseng roots stand alone in their class.

Wild ginseng is the highest-priced North American product, while ginseng cultivated under artificial shade is the lowest-priced root. The differences in appearance are striking. Dried wild roots are generally smaller than a man's thumb, feather light, well ringed, and dark tan to light brown in color. Field-cultivated roots are large, disproportionately heavy, poorly ringed, and straw colored. The important distinction for growers is the market price. Field-cultivated roots bring a mere 15 to 30 percent of the price of wild roots. Only natural shade produces roots exhibiting characteristics of the more valuable wild roots. While all of these cultivation methods are discussed in this book, entrepreneurs entering today's competitive ginseng market would do well to consider natural-shade production and the quality root it produces.

Chapter 1

Ginseng Species

America became a commercial rival to Chos-en as early as 1757, when the products of Connecticut and Massachusetts lay side by side with Corean [Korean] imports in the markets of Peking and Canton.

Corea, *The Hermit Nation,*
William Elliot Griffis
New York, 1904

Several species of ginseng exist within the Araliaceae family and the genus *Panax*. Most exhibit medicinal properties, but interestingly, each species has a different chemical makeup and has a unique application in traditional Chinese medicine. In general, all true ginseng contains biologically active saponins, essential oil, phytosterol, carbohydrates, sugars, organic acids, nitrogenous substances, amino acids, peptides, vitamins, and minerals. More and more Western researchers are taking a serious look at ginseng in a variety of experiments, from lowering cholesterol to maintaining metabolic balance during the treatment of AIDS.

AMERICAN GINSENG

Wild American ginseng, *Panax quinquefolium,* is indigenous to southern Canada and the eastern and midwestern United States. It has historically been found between thirty and fifty degrees north latitude, encompassing portions of thirty-four U.S. states. In Canada the natural range of wild ginseng is much more modest, only extending eastward from the Great Lakes region south of the fiftieth parallel. First discovered in 1716 by a Jesuit priest, American ginseng can still be found in porous, well-drained loam soil throughout the mountains and river bluffs of eastern North America. The plant requires a canopy of shade that filters approximately 78 percent of the direct sunlight.

Ginseng is an erect perennial plant that rarely exceeds twenty-four inches in height. Ginseng native to southern states tends to have purplish stalks, while northern ginseng only has tinges of purple on green stems. Southern ginseng also emerges in the spring without a visible flower stem, while northern plants have a fully developed flower peduncle between the leaves when they emerge.

Ginseng has three or four compound leaves arranged in a whorl when mature, each leaf containing five ovate, saw-toothed

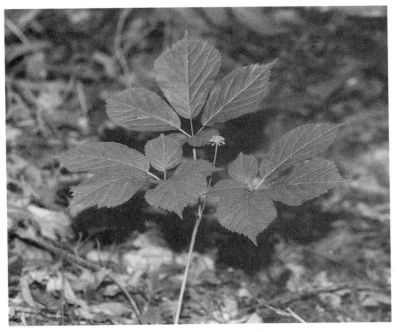

Wild American ginseng in June

leaflets. The upper three leaflets are larger than the lower two. The leaves are referred to as prongs; thus, a ginseng plant with three leaves (and five leaflets on each leaf) would be called a three-pronger. In its immature form, ginseng is only a one- or two-pronger. During the first growing season, ginseng has a single three- to four-inch stem with three leaflets and looks more like poison ivy than a mature ginseng plant.

A ginseng plant adds an additional leaf every few years until it achieves its mature leaf arrangement of three prongs. Since it competes with a number of other forest plants for nutrients, this process is excruciatingly slow. Native plants may not become three-prongers for ten years or more. Older wild plants will have four prongs, but due to heavy digging pressure throughout much of the range, three are more common. Field-cultivated ginseng plants routinely produce four prongs within four or five years.

Ginseng is found naturally in forested areas with a pH of 5.5 to 6.5 and annual precipitation of twenty to sixty inches. It grows very slowly and is extremely long-lived. Plants over one hundred years old have been reported. For example, a one-hundred-year-old Asian ginseng root was discovered in 1981 in the Jangbaeck Mountain Range in China. Most of the older wild roots (both American and Asian) have been dug over the years, however, and today's forager can expect to find roots between twelve and twenty years old. Thirty- or forty-year-old roots might still be found, but they are becoming increasingly uncommon.

The growing season for ginseng is late April or early May through late September or early October across its range. In general, the older plants will sprout first each spring, with each younger year class emerging five days or so after the last. Under natural shade, the plants do not follow this sequence exactly because of variances in soil temperatures. Still, the one- and two-year-olds can be expected to sprout a week to ten days after the older plants.

Plants in the southern range will sprout earlier and die down later than plants in the northern range because of the greater number of frost-free days in the South. There is little correlation, however, between the number of frost-free days and the actual growth of the ginseng root. Roots grow best in cool soil, and the long, hot summer days of the South actually inhibit root growth. The cooler weather of the northern states allows the ginseng root to maintain slow but steady growth right through the summer. Roots from southern states tend to grow rapidly for a few weeks in the spring and then level off throughout the warmer months with little appreciable weight gain. Northern and southern roots both show a growth spurt after the berries ripen.

Seed production tasks the plants throughout the summer, starting with the greenish-white flowers that appear on a flower stem rising from the center of the whorl of prongs. The ginseng plant is self-pollinating, but nature provides some cross-pollination by way of sweat bees (halictid bees). These tiny bees can be seen busily buzzing from plant to plant as long as flowers remain. Hover flies also pollinate ginseng flowers, although to a much lesser degree than the sweat bees. Common honeybees can occasionally be seen visiting ginseng patches. Thick stands of cultivated ginseng seem to have no need for the tiny pollinators, but the insects may be of assistance to wild and wild-simulated plants. Some cross-pollination likely provides offspring of good genetic strength.

The tiny ginseng flowers quickly swell into small green, kidney-shaped berries that ripen to a brilliant crimson color from early August until diedown. The seeds do not all ripen at once, so plants with ripe red berries can be found side by side with those having full-size green berries and others not far beyond the flowering state. Perhaps some genetic encoding compels plants in a patch to act this way, attracting seed-gathering birds and rodents for many weeks.

As the berries ripen, they draw animals that feast on the seeds inside the bitter, crimson fruits. Each berry contains one to three seeds, and a few seeds will be scattered as the predator nibbles on the others. Chipmunks and mice are particularly fond of ginseng seeds and can sometimes be seen trying to drag an entire seed head into a thicket, where the seeds can be consumed at leisure. This actually aids the ginseng population, because a few seeds invariably drop and find their way between tiny rock crevices or under twigs and fallen branches, where they will lie for eighteen months of dormancy. Birds also eat the berries and expel the seeds in their droppings after digesting the pulp. Some old-time diggers claim that ginseng seeds germinate best if they've been "run through a bird first." Patches of wild ginseng are often found in grapevine thickets where ruffed grouse or wild turkeys take refuge.

Ginseng seeds do not sprout the first spring after ripening but wait until the second spring. This eighteen- to twenty-month dormant period allows the imperfect embryo inside the shell to fully develop before emerging. During this span, the seeds must remain moist to be viable. Drying to more than half their weight will kill the tiny seeds, and they will rattle if shaken. Fallen leaves from deciduous trees provide a natural blanket over the seeds each autumn, but an extended dry spell during the late summer and early autumn months can spell doom for partially exposed seeds. During the eighteen-month dormant period, many dangers stalk the tiny ginseng seeds. Rodents are always on the lookout for the tasty morsels. Moles, through their burrowing action, can push the seeds deep into the soil, where they become hopelessly bound and die.

After the seeds are produced and dispersed, the ginseng plant prepares itself for a winter dormant period. The bud atop the "neck" of the root swells rapidly and the root itself goes through a growth spurt, concentrating sugars and saponins in preparation for the high-stress period the next spring when it will push another plant toward the heavens. As energy is stored in the root and photosynthesis stops, the leaves turn a droopy yellow, eventually falling away from the main stem in the brisk autumn winds. The stem remains the longest and indeed may survive for an entire year, standing in a poignantly stiff, wilted state alongside the new growth of the next year. Veteran ginseng diggers, called 'sangers, keep an eye out for dried stalks jutting from the ground when they find a patch of ginseng, since ginseng sometimes "skips a year" in sending up a new plant. Digging around a wilted stalk can reveal a healthy ginseng root, apparently dormant, saving its energy for a full year before producing a new plant. The reason for this dormancy is not known, but it may be that the root does not always have enough nutrients to produce a plant each year. Or perhaps some behavioral encoding prompts the root to use this tactic as protection against predators. The odd phenomenon has likely saved many a ginseng plant from diggers who missed the root because it was tucked safely underground with no visible leaves during the digging season.

The ginseng root is fleshy, aromatic, and spindle shaped, looking somewhat like a small, distorted carrot. It has a mildly bitter taste. Ginseng diggers often chew on a root while hiking the hills in search of the wild plants because they say it gives them energy. The mature ginseng root is generally forked and has a tendency to branch into a number of odd shapes.

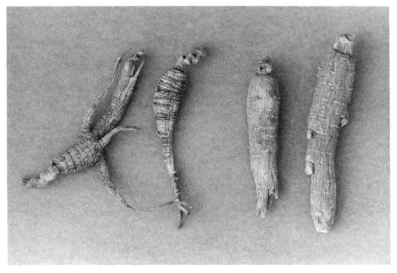

Ginseng roots: wild (left) and cultivated (right)

The interior of the root is creamy-white and will remain so during proper drying. The skin has a golden tint and will dry to a golden brown color, although the character of the local soil can affect the root's exterior color. Ginseng is not a spreading rhizome, and it usually sprouts a single plant from the top of the neck each year. Strong roots will occasionally have two necks, and subsequently support two plants, but one is more common. In rare instances wild ginseng can be found with three or more stalks arising from a single, massive root.

During the summer, a small bud appears on the root beside the current year's plant. Each year this bud appears atop the scar left by the previous plant and eventually develops the next year's plant. These cup-shaped bud scars build a neck that actually tells the plant's age. Each scar represents one year's growth, so counting the bud scars on the neck will reveal the age of the root. If the neck is broken, however, the root will form a new bud immediately atop the broken neck, thereby "losing" the amount of scars that have been become detached. In this case, the age cannot be determined accurately. The neck sometimes develops blight and rots away completely. If the rot does not spread to the main root, a new bud will form near the top of the unaffected section of root and begin a new neck. Ginseng's characteristic neck allows the root to take on a personlike appearance. Roots with a human appearance were considered superior at one time, but that no longer holds true.

The mature root is prominently marked on the outside with rings similar to the spirals on a screw. These markings are indicative of a long, slow growth under stress and add to the value of the root. Wild ginseng roots have this important characteristic. Most cultivated roots are not well ringed, and this lowers their value dramatically.

The Koreans theorize that the ginseng root contracts in September or October of each year and actually "wriggles" deeper into the soil to accommodate the upward growth of the neck. The yearly shrinking of the root keeps the bud stem underground and helps to produce the valuable circles or transverse wrinkles around the root. The theory would seem to have merit, because the neck of the ginseng root rarely protrudes about the soil surface, no matter how elongated it has become.

A close relative of American ginseng, *Panax trifolious,* or dwarf ginseng, can be found across the eastern United States. Dwarf ginseng has no medicinal or commercial value and is somewhat rare.

Another ginseng relative commonly seen in eastern woodlands is wild sarsaparilla, *Aralia nudicaulis.* The wild sarsaparilla plant closely resembles American ginseng and is frequently mistaken by novice foragers as true ginseng. Because of this, wild sarsaparilla is known as "fool's 'sang." It can be distinguished from the ginseng plant by its detached leaflet arrangement; the upper three leaflets do not meet the lower two on the leaf stem. Wild sarsaparilla's rootstock is a long rhizome that snakes along just below the soil surface. This is quite unlike ginseng's stocky, deep-rooted tuber. Wild sarsaparilla is occasionally found in the vicinity of ginseng, but it usually prefers a drier soil than ginseng.

Quite a few other wild plants are companions to ginseng in its natural habitat. Called "good weeds" by Appalachian 'sangers, these companion plants include Indian turnip (jack-in-the-pulpit), black cohosh, blue cohosh, goldenseal, and bloodroot. Several of these plants have low-grade medicinal values, but they are rarely harvested. Goldenseal is the exception. It is worth digging at $20 per pound. Christmas ferns can be good indicators that ginseng is nearby, but most ferns are not. Veteran 'sangers always look for good weeds when scouting new ginseng habitat. This forest vegetation is also useful to the woodland cultivator as an indicator of good ginseng soil.

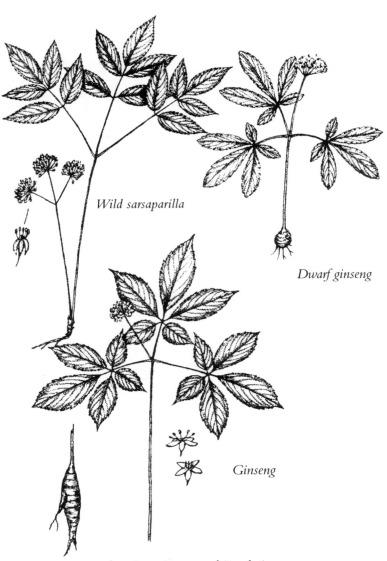

Wild sarsaparilla

Dwarf ginseng

Ginseng

American ginseng and its relatives

ASIAN GINSENG

Asian ginseng, *Panax ginseng* (Carl Anton Meyer, 1843) or *Panax shinseng* (Nees van Esenbeck, 1833), is native to a series of mountain ranges in Manchuria, China, Korea, and several of the newly independent states of the former Soviet Union. As with the North American variety, Asian ginseng occurs between thirty and fifty degrees north latitude. Although on the brink of extinction, wild Asian ginseng is still being hunted by the Chinese, North Koreans, and Siberian Russians. About eighty pounds of wild Asian ginseng are harvested annually in that region of the world. These highly prized roots of "imperial ginseng" command the exorbitant price of $55,000 per pound, making them the most valuable raw herbs in the world. Cultivated Asian ginseng is much lower in price.

The Asian plant is similar to American ginseng, although it is slightly more slender and elongated in appearance. Some Asian plants produce yellow berries instead of the usual crimson, a phenomenon completely unknown in the American species. The Asian seeds have a slightly rougher texture than seeds from American plants. Ginseng habitat in the Orient is quite like that of American ginseng. An observer walking through a deciduous forest of northern China might very well mistake his or her surroundings for that of a pleasant Wisconsin woodland.

Asiatic ginseng is recognized in several varieties in addition to the authentic *Panax ginseng*. These include *Panax notoginseng* (Burk), known as sanchi or tienchi ginseng, from China; *Panax pseudoginseng* (Wall) from Afghanistan's Hindu Kush mountains, Nepal, and the eastern Himalayas; and *Panax japonicus* (Meyer), or bamboo ginseng, from Japan. These are generally considered as a species separate from the more valuable *Panax ginseng*. All are graded quite differently by ginseng merchants. Native Japanese

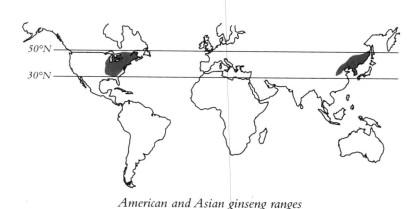

American and Asian ginseng ranges

ginseng is considered the lowest-quality ginseng in the world, perhaps due to the rocky, alkaline soil there. The Japanese have imported Korean seed and are now cultivating that variety instead of their native stock.

OTHER MEDICINAL RELATIVES

Siberian ginseng, *Eleutherococcus senticosus,* is not really a ginseng at all, but a cousin within the Araliaceae family. Also known as eleuthero ginseng and devil's shrub, it has a long history of use within certain regions of China, while in other areas it is looked upon with disdain. More recent Soviet research has catapulted it into worldwide scrutiny as an adaptogen to stressful conditions. It is much more widely distributed in the Orient than the true ginseng, ranging across parts of the former Soviet Union, China, Korea, and Japan.

A shrubby forest plant with spine-laced stalks, Siberian ginseng reaches a height of eight to ten feet and can form nearly impenetrable thickets. Test plots have been established in the northwestern United States from imported seeds. It is not a competitor of American ginseng.

Chapter 2

History of American Ginseng

If ginseng is to be found in any other region of the world, it may be particularly in Canada, where the forest and mountains, according to those who have lived there, are very much like those of China.

Father Pierre Jartoux,
Jesuit missionary to China,
Peking, 12 April 1711

The Jesuit priests who roamed the known world in the seventeenth and eighteenth centuries were not only missionaries but also explorers held in high esteem throughout the scientific community. These priest-adventurers conducted lengthy studies on plants and animals encountered in exotic lands. Their findings were circulated in dispatches around the globe so that priests in desolate or remote posts could keep up with news about their comrades. In 1716, Father Joseph Francois Lafitau (1681–1746), a Jesuit priest in Canada, read Jartoux's manuscripts from the Orient in which ginseng was described in minute detail. Determined to find a similar herb around the Suzanne Creek Mission (near Montreal) to which he was assigned, Lafitau set about searching the forests in hopes of locating an American variety of the man-root.

Some stories allege that the Mohawk Indians of the Iroquois Six Nations helped the priest ferret out the plant they called *garantoquen,* but Lafitau's translation of the word *ginseng* from French into Native American tongues probably did nothing but confuse the Mohawks as to which of their myriad of medicinal plants Lafitau was trying to find. It is therefore generally accepted that Lafitau actually discovered American ginseng by his own hand. Interestingly, the contents of one of his letters supports this supposition, describing the discovery of New World ginseng thus:

Having spent three months searching for ginseng to no avail, I found it quite by accident when I was not thinking of it at all, near a house I was having built. It was in fruit and the bright red berries caught my eye. The first sight of it made me think this might be the plant I was seeking. I pulled it up without delay and carried it off joyfully to a native woman whom I had employed to look for it. She recognized it immediately as one of their ordinary remedies and described its uses.

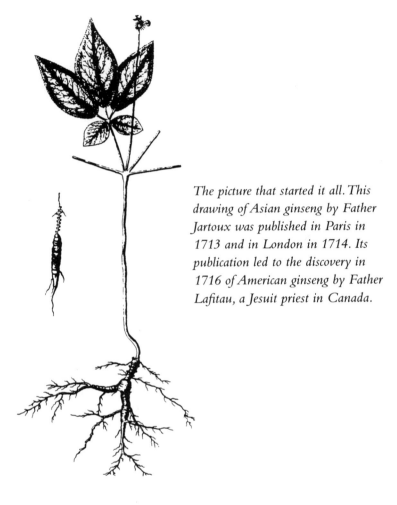

The picture that started it all. This drawing of Asian ginseng by Father Jartoux was published in Paris in 1713 and in London in 1714. Its publication led to the discovery in 1716 of American ginseng by Father Lafitau, a Jesuit priest in Canada.

The letter goes on for several pages describing Lafitau's surprise in learning that the Mohawk word for ginseng, *garantoquen,* meant man's thighs, or more generally, man's image. He considered this remarkable analogue to the Chinese translation of man-root to be more than a coincidence and wrote:

I could only conclude that the same meaning could not have been applied in the Chinese and Iroquois words without a communication of ideas, and by consequence of persons. By this I confirmed an opinion which I already had, which is based on other judgments, that America made one continent with Asia, united at Tartary to the north of China.

The theory of an ancient land bridge between Asia and North America at the Bering Strait is now widely accepted within the scientific community, but three hundred years ago it must have been an extraordinary concept. Lafitau's insight in associating a common ancestry between Asians and Native Americans is all the more interesting when we realize that it is based, in large part, on the discovery of ginseng on the North American continent.

Within a few years of American ginseng's discovery, French-Canadian traders and Indians were gathering the roots for export to China. By the mid-1700s, a sizeable ginseng export business had sprung up. But disaster struck when a large shipment of poorly harvested and improperly dried roots reached China. The Chinese merchants refused to purchase any more French-Canadian ginseng, and the ginseng business of our northern neighbors collapsed. Luck was with them in a way, since the unrestricted harvest of immature plants had severely decimated Canada's wild ginseng population. The forced respite from digging allowed the plant to totter back from the brink of extinction in that country.

The search for forest gold soon spread into the British colonies to the south. By 1757, ships loaded with ginseng were plying down the Hudson River heading for Amsterdam and London, where European middlemen raked in huge profits from commerce with China. Over the years, this indirect trade through the "Sovereign Crown" and the taxation on tea returning from the Orient caused considerable resentment among the American colonists. Samuel Shaw, a colonial patriot, stated, "The Americans must have tea, and they seek the most lucrative market for their precious root ginseng."

The American-Chinese trade began in earnest after the Revolutionary War. One of the first American ships to transport ginseng directly from the new United States of America to China was the *Empress of China,* under the command of Captain John Greene. The supercargo (master of cargo) on board was none other than Samuel Shaw. The *Empress of China* sailed south from New York on February 22, 1784, rounded Cape Horn, crossed the broad expanse of the Pacific Ocean, and made port in Canton on August 30, 1784. A profit of 30 percent was realized from this six-month venture, and colonists were prodded to brave the dangers of the western wilderness in order to bring more of the valuable roots to market.

The exploration of the Northwest territories (the region west of Pennsylvania) was under way at this time, and ginseng was found there in profusion. Exploitation of the unblemished land's riches was inevitable. 'Sangers set pick and shovel to ginseng patches that blanketed the forest. Some patches covered acres, and the diggers often camped in the middle of a patch until they had dug it all. John Mathews, surveyor for the Ohio Land Company, casually described the glut of ginseng in Ohio's Muskingum River Valley in his diary entry of September 22, 1787:

> Left our camp at sunrise and moved about five miles to the west and encamped about half a mile to the east of the dividing ridge between the waters of Muskingum and Short creek. Here we dug ginseng until Thursday, 27th. It grew in great abundance. Men accustomed to the work could dig from forty to sixty pounds a day.

Before the turn of the century, many thousands of pounds of ginseng roots were harvested in the Northwest Territories and shipped east for exportation to the Orient. Daniel Boone (1734–1820) was one of the more famous colonist trailblazers to engage in the ginseng trade. After the Revolutionary War, Colonel Boone turned to commerce and decided he could make a handsome profit in ginseng. In 1787 he and several hired hands set about digging all the ginseng they could find along the ridges of western Virginia (now West Virginia) and eastern Kentucky. Boone also bought roots from other 'sangers and eventually amassed a fifteen-ton cache of forest gold. The following spring he loaded a boat and headed up the Ohio River for Pittsburgh, from whence the roots would be shipped overland to Philadelphia. But calamity struck before he made port in Pennsylvania: His boat sank in shallow water at the head of an island near Point Pleasant, West Virginia, soaking his valuable cargo. Boone was able to recover part of his shipment and send it on to Philadelphia, but the delay and water damage cost him dearly. His cargo arrived on the East Coast just as the price of ginseng dropped, and the damaged roots brought very little of what the Chinese were then offering.

In a subsequent letter to a friend, Boone commented, "I cannot help reflecting a litel on the downfall of ginsagn wch ware a litel unfortenit last fall but I doubt it will be worse this." Undaunted, he set out to gather more ginseng and experienced considerable success in the ginseng trade during later years.

John Jacob Astor of the American Fur Company was another early American who successfully speculated in the ginseng trade. Born in Germany, he moved to London and there became involved in the fur trade before emigrating to America in 1784. Teaming up with New York shipowner John Livermore, Astor shrewdly bought all the ginseng he could lay his hands on and sent a shipload of roots off to China. Many months later the ship returned to New York with valuable Chinese tea and Astor's share of the ginseng profits—$55,000 in silver! Astor's road to fortune was, at least initially, paved with ginseng roots.

The digging of wild ginseng continued unabated into and throughout the 1800s. Records indicate that perhaps twenty million pounds of dried wild ginseng roots were shipped from the United States to China from the end of the Revolutionary War until 1900. Considering the minimum green-to-dry weight ratio of three to one, more than sixty million pounds of America's forest gold were dug in about 120 years!

The exploitation of American ginseng could not last. By the end of the Civil War ginseng had become scarce in parts of its natural range. Thoughts turned to cultivation of the valuable root, but most attempts failed. The early cultivators often used improper shade or no shade at all and were beset by disease. Around 1885, George Stanton pioneered ginseng cultivation in the United States. A tinsmith by trade, Stanton was also known as a rather ingenious individual who had several patents recorded in his name. He eventually gave up his tin business because of poor health and turned to ginseng culture as a less strenuous undertaking. The George Stanton Chinese Ginseng Farm became his life's work. His experiments in ginseng culture eventually showed that ginseng could be "tamed" and interested others in ginseng cultivation as a profitable enterprise. By the time of his death on January 31, 1908, Stanton had been honored by his peers with the title Father of the Ginseng Industry.

Ginseng cultivation had its ups and downs over the ensuing century, with many gardens being wiped out in the early 1900s by Alternaria blight. This was the low point in U.S. cultivation. The introduction of an effective fungicide, Bordeaux mixture, improved matters, and cultivators once more entered the business. Most, however, found that ginseng was not an overnight road to riches as they had been led to believe. Long years of wait loomed ahead for the ginseng entrepreneur before a harvest, and pests, disease, and theft could wipe out a ginseng farm in a few short days.

During World War II, most of the ginseng growers east of Wisconsin, mainly in New York, Pennsylvania, Ohio, and Indiana, went out of business. From 1940 to 1947 the Japanese occupied the Chinese coastline and stopped ginseng exports to mainland China. With the market in a state of collapse, only a few major growers around Wausau, Wisconsin, remained in the business. After 1947 the demand for both wild and cultivated American ginseng increased by 25 to 30 percent annually. Those Wisconsin growers who had toughed out the eight lean years went on to establish Wisconsin as the center of cultivated ginseng in the United States. Today, Wisconsin farms produce about 99 percent of all the cultivated ginseng grown in the United States.

Although cultivated roots make up the bulk of America's ginseng exports, wild ginseng continues to be dug and sold in many states. The harvest of wild ginseng has remained fairly constant over the past few years because of government regulation. As a signatory to CITIES, the Convention on International Trade in Endangered Species of Flora and Fauna, the U.S. government is committed to protecting ginseng in this country. Under the terms of CITIES, the U.S. Fish and Wildlife Service monitors ginseng populations here and restricts international trade in the roots in order to ensure the continued survival of American ginseng.

Currently, ginseng is listed on CITIES Appendix II, which means international trade is allowed under controlled conditions. Wild and cultivated ginseng are considered the same species under this treaty. The Federal Wildlife Permit Office therefore issues import and export permits for both wild and cultivated ginseng.

States must develop regulations acceptable to the USFWS that demonstrate reasonable protection for ginseng within their borders. States that do not comply cannot export ginseng.

Regulations for wild ginseng generally include an open digging season after the berries have ripened, a stipulation that immature plants cannot be harvested, and a requirement that berries from harvested mature plants be planted in the same vicinity as the parent plant. A permit is always required to ship ginseng roots out of state, and in some instances the digger needs a state permit in order to hunt for ginseng.

Like hunting or fishing regulations, the laws vary slightly in each state, so diggers and growers should contact the agency responsible for ginseng protection in their state, often the state forestry or wildlife agency. Anyone interested in digging wild ginseng is strongly urged to follow all of the conservation practices in effect in his or her region.

Ginseng has been recognized as an important part of Americana. It helped support our fledgling nation in its fight for independence and opened the vast American wilderness to exploration. Today it reduces our nation's trade deficit and shows promise in the treatment of a number of modern ailments. Ginseng has been, and is destined to remain, a viable and fruitful part of our national heritage.

Chapter 3

The Legendary
Ginseng Root

In the province of Leotung a root is produced which is sold at the price of double its weight in silver. It is a marvelous medicine, which is able to increase the strength of the frame and to restore the exhausted animal powers. The Chinese call it gin sem.

The earliest published mention
of ginseng in Europe,
Alvaro Semmedo,
Rome, 1643

Shen Nung, the second emperor of the "Three August Rulers" is credited with being China's "Divine Farmer," or the father of agriculture and herbal therapy. Nearly five thousand years ago he compiled China's first detailed description of drugs and medicine into a pharmacopoeia called the *Pen Ts'ao*. In it, ginseng is rated as the most potent herbal remedy known to man. Records from this era are rather unclear, so it is not known whether this information was passed down through the generations verbally or in some written form. What is known is that during the first century A.D., and again several times over the ensuing Chinese dynasties, the work was compiled and credited to Shen Nung. Some editions are referred to as the *Materia Medica* in addition to *Pen Ts'ao*. The current *Pen Ts'ao Kung Mu,* written during the 16th century by Li Shi-Chen (whose name is also translated into English as ShiZhen Li, 1518–1593 A.D.), is a massive assembly of historical herbal remedies, many of which are still in use today.

Ginseng is historically linked with China, but it was known on the ancient Indian continent as well. The famous *Artharva Veda* of India proclaims:

> [Ginseng] aids in bringing forth the seed that is poured into the female that forsooth is the way to bring forth a son . . . the strength of the horse, the mule, the goat and the ram, moreover the strength of the bull ginseng bestows on him. This herb will make thee so full of lusty strength that thou shalt, when thou art excited, exhale heat as a thing on fire.

The French Jesuit priest Jartoux, a trained cartographer assigned to Peking in 1709, set down a careful description and drawing of Asian ginseng in a 1711 correspondence to the Procurator General of the Missions of India and China. Entitled "The Description of a

Tartarian Plant, called Gin-seng: with an Account of its Virtues," this letter received wide translation and recognition in Europe. In it Jartoux reports:

> The most eminent physicians in China . . . affirm that ginseng is a sovereign remedy for all weaknesses occasioned by excessive fatigues either of body or mind, that it dissolves pituitous humors, that it cures weakness of the lungs and pleurisy, that it stops vomiting, that it strengthens the stomach and helps the appetite, that it disperses fumes or vapors, that it fortifies the breast, and is a remedy for short or weak breathing, that it strengthens the vital spirits and increases lymph in the blood, in short, that it is good against dizziness of the head and dimness of sight, and that it prolongs life in old age. Nobody can imagine that the Chinese and Tartars would set so high a value upon this root if it did not constantly produce a good effect.

Father Jartoux also described his chance meeting with a group of ginseng hunters sent out by the emperor to gather ginseng roots in the wilderness of Tartary (northeastern China). The terrain was characterized by Jartoux as "a long tract of mountains covered and encompassed by thick forests that render them almost unpassable." The hunters' promised reward was to make a gift of two ounces of their best roots to the emperor and receive payment for the balance in fine silver according to its weight. For this, Father Jartoux noted, they braved frightful perils:

> These poor people suffer a great deal in this expedition. They carry with them neither tents nor beds, everyone being sufficiently loaded with his provisions, which is

only millet parched in an oven, upon which he must subsist all the time of his journey. They are constrained to sleep under trees, having only their branches and barks, if they can find them, for their covering. Their mandarins send them from time to time pieces of beef, or such game as they happen to take, which they eat greedily and almost raw. If any one of them is wanting, as it often happens, either by wandering out of the way, or being devoured by wild beasts, they look for him a day or two, and then return again to their labor as before.

Jartoux's letter eventually made its way to publication in 1713. This dispatch was read by Father Lafitau half a world away several years later and led to the European discovery of American ginseng.

Ginseng's discovery in the New World paved the way for an international market with the Far East. Today the ginseng trade remains a profitable endeavor, with the United States exporting ginseng worth $100 million a year. The roots from the modern American ginseng farm are still graded much the same as they were during the remote Chinese dynasties—according to their physical attributes and not on their pharmacological qualities:

Size	the bigger the better
Shape	the thicker the better
Age	the older the better
Rings	the more the better
Texture	the coarser the better
Color (exterior)	golden brown to dark brown with no rust or rot
Color (interior)	creamy-white interior when trimmed

The ideal that is strived for is an old wild root. It will be plump with a long neck, will be heavily ringed, and will feel as light as a cork. W. W. Stockberger's comments in the 1921 edition of *Ginseng Culture, Farmer's Bulletin No. 1184* still ring true today:

> Growers should strive for quality of product and not for quantity of production, as has been the all too common practice in the past. There is always a ready sale for the cultivated roots which closely resemble the wild in quality and condition, and prudent growers will not fail to adopt the wild root as the standard of future production.

American ginseng roots are broadly graded as field-cultivated (under an artificial shade canopy), woodsgrown, wild-simulated, and wild. Field-cultivated ginseng exhibits the least desirable qualities and brings the lowest price. Wild is the ideal root and fetches the premium price. Woodsgrown and wild-simulated roots lie somewhere in between. Cultivation methods for each grade of root are discussed in this book, but the emphasis is on woodsgrown and wild-simulated ginseng. The Canadians are rapidly expanding their artificial-shade production and will be pumping several hundred thousand additional pounds of low-grade roots into the market within a few years. Prices for field-cultivated roots may fall when these roots hit the market. But maturing markets in Malaysia and Singapore, where American wild ginseng is at a premium, will produce a heavy demand for wild or near-wild roots. Since the harvest of wild roots has remained fairly constant for the past five years and is not expected to increase, the cultivator who provides this type of root will find a great demand for his product over the next few decades. So let's grow some ginseng!

Chapter 4

Ginseng Cultivation

Ginseng is truly and wholly a savage . . . it cannot be greatly changed from its nature without suffering the consequences.

Ginseng and Other Medicinal Plants,
A. R. Harding
1908

Although early growers encountered seemingly insurmountable problems in transferring ginseng from the forest to the garden, ginseng can now be successfully cultivated in many areas outside of its natural range, as long as its native habitat is approximated. Here in the United States, ginseng farms have sprung up in the Pacific Northwest and several other areas far removed from ginseng's eastern origin. Northern climates are favored, since ginseng needs a minimum cold cycle of sixty days with temperatures below forty-nine degrees Fahrenheit (or forty-five days with temperatures below thirty-six degrees Fahrenheit) in order to break dormancy each spring. Rainfall of twenty to sixty inches per year is the plant's natural requirement. Loam topsoil, light in texture, well drained with organic material and slightly acidic properties, is ideal. Heavy clay or very sandy soils are not suitable for ginseng cultivation. Although a big chunk of the country has less-than-perfect growing conditions for ginseng, a determined grower with some ingenuity and a little luck may be able to tackle borderline tracts and come out ahead. If you live in marginal growing regions, start small and be prepared for many trial-and-error learning experiences.

One item is essential for ginseng cultivation anywhere in the world: shade. Like any other green plant, ginseng requires sunlight, but because it's a forest plant, it needs shade, too. No amount of "taming" has yet yielded a ginseng plant that can withstand direct sunlight.

Three distinct cultivation methods for American ginseng are recognized, under two types of shade. Net return under a particular method varies with the initial investment and the age of the roots at harvest.

Field cultivation under artificial shade gives the highest yield per acre but also takes the largest investment of time and money. Up-front costs for land, seed, shade, machinery, and labor run $30,000 to $35,000 per acre. Gross returns per acre run as high as

$100,000 after four years. Field-cultivated ginseng is the lowest grade of ginseng, currently priced at $25 to $50 per pound, dried weight.

Woodsgrown ginseng is raised under a natural tree canopy in a forest setting. Some maintenance is required, and intensive cultivation methods may be used to maximize yields in minimal time. Investment costs are markedly lower for woodsgrown ginseng because the shade is provided by nature and less machinery is used. Applications of pesticides and fertilizer are generally, but not always, reduced. The value of woodsgrown ginseng varies considerably, since the finished product may resemble field-cultivated at one extreme and the more precious wild-simulated at the other. The five- to eight-year wait until harvest is longer than for field-cultivated ginseng but shorter than for wild-simulated roots. Prices fluctuate with the quality of the root produced, but growers can receive $20 to $40 more per pound for woodsgrown ginseng than for field-cultivated roots. If the roots resemble the more valuable wild-simulated ginseng, the price can go much higher.

Like woodsgrown ginseng, wild-simulated ginseng is grown under a natural shade canopy, but very little attention is paid to the plants after seeding. Light maintenance, such as weeding and a minimal use of pesticides or fungicides may be undertaken, but the plants are essentially left to fend for themselves. Investment costs are low and returns high since the roots will resemble the extremely valuable wild ginseng. The time from planting to harvest is quite long, averaging ten to fifteen years. After ten years, you should receive a price close to that for wild roots.

All three methods have their pros and cons. A big initial investment and forty-plus hours a week will reap you a nice return in a relatively short time under artificial shade. If you're not looking for a major investment and a full-time job, woodsgrown or wild-simulated may be the better choice. Although the time to harvest is the longest for wild-simulated, your patience can produce a long-term yield that has the potential to top anything in your investment portfolio.

PLANNING THE GINSENG GARDEN

Ginseng farming requires a plan, whether it be for a multiacre endeavor under artificial shade or a widely scattered planting under natural shade conditions. Economics are, of course, a major factor to consider in ginseng cultivation. From a hobby-type enterprise of one tenth of an acre, to a side business encompassing an acre or so, to a major undertaking of many acres, investment funds and potential yields are the driving forces.

What can you expect to make from your investment in seed, material, fertilizers, sprays, equipment usage, and time? A very rough guideline is $1,000 gross return per pound of seed planted. Initial purchases of seed (fluctuating between $60 and over $100 per pound at this writing) can absorb quite a bit of your potential profit. As your garden matures and produces seed, however, this expense is reduced or eliminated.

Artificial shade requires a considerable investment in material, time, and labor. For example, material costs are currently about $8,000 per acre for fabric shade, cables, connectors, and posts. Initial labor costs must be assessed, since one or two people would be hard-pressed to handle a large-scale setup—fifty clamps alone weigh 68 pounds, and five thousand feet of cable tip the scale at 640 pounds. Tractors, plows, bed-makers, and diggers are additional expenses to be considered. But the special machinery and material can be reused for many years, reducing future cash outlays for new acres planted. Luckily, initial investment costs for ginseng grown under natural shade are less than half that of artificial shade plantings.

No matter what your method of cultivation or initial investment, time is an important factor. Ginseng roots cannot be harvested until they are three to four years old under artificial shade, and it may take up to fifteen years to grow a marketable root under natural shade.

As you can see, the business of ginseng is not quite so simple as shoving a few seeds into the ground and growing gold. Optimism and operating capital are basic qualifications for the job. Still, a ginseng venture can be quite profitable if a solid plan is developed and followed.

The techniques used for field-cultivated ginseng are very intensive, and many can be adapted to natural-shade cultivation. The specifics of machinery will not be discussed in depth here because farmers and gardeners are more likely to adapt their own equipment than buy commercially available machinery or conversions, at least for their initial plots.

If you intend to make ginseng cultivation your life's work, research the industry before taking the plunge. A tour of a working ginseng farm is a good idea. Take note of the equipment and machinery in use and ask lots of questions. If you want to grow ginseng as a hobby, an investment, or part of a retirement strategy, you will also find a farm visit useful and inspiring. Some of the sources for seeds and roots listed in the Appendix may permit tours of their gardens.

Work on a ginseng garden begins well in advance of the autumn planting date. Most commercial growers plot out and start working their gardens one and a half years prior to planting. Brush and small trees must be cleared on forest sites, leaving only enough mature trees to give sufficient shade. Cleaning out the lower trees and limbs is vitally important for good air circulation throughout the garden. Soil tests are done and amendments added. The area is tilled several times in the year preceding planting in order to work the ground and kill weeds that sprout.

Walking the future site immediately after a heavy rain can help the cultivator detect areas with poor drainage. These spots are then marked and avoided, or raised beds are put in place. An eye must also be kept on the shade, since a windstorm can fell trees and leave gaps in the natural shade. Adjustments can be made in the expected planting zones or plans can be devised to temporarily cover the openings with artificial shade.

Another consideration is previous ginseng plantings in the area. Ginseng can never be grown twice on the same land under artificial shade because the soil pathogens build to such a high level during the first ginseng crop that a second crop simply cannot survive four years for a second harvest. Commercial farmers who have attempted to grow ginseng in previously used ginseng fields report that most of the plants die by the third year. Ginseng can follow other crops, such as corn and alfalfa, but only if ginseng has not already been grown in that field.

The growers of Wisconsin's Marathon County keep close track of the ginseng fields in production each year so that they don't rent a farm that has already had ginseng planted on it. As you might expect, ginseng farmers employing artificial shade become fairly mobile, since new fields must be purchased or rented each year to stay in business. It is thought that letting the land lie idle for fifteen or more years may reduce the soilborne pathogens enough to permit a second ginseng harvest, but there have been no definitive studies in this area.

Woodland gardens are usually not plagued with this "once and done" handicap, but the wise grower will not tempt fate by making two consecutive plantings in the same beds. A fallow period of several years is a good bet before reseeding under natural shade. Wild-simulated plantings seem not to be affected in the least by this problem. The small patches probably never build up enough pathogens to seriously endanger subsequent seedings.

SHADE

The first major decision facing today's ginseng farmer is what type of shade to use. Like most small- to moderate-plot growers, I consider natural shade superior for quality production. It takes a lot longer to get a harvest, but the investment is fairly low and you can't beat the top-notch roots. Artificial shade will give you a hefty harvest of low-grade roots—more pounds per acre than you could ever hope to grow under natural shade—but you constantly worry about whether the shade will blow away in heavy weather, if you need to spray after every rain, if the drainage is okay, how much it will cost to have the weeds picked, and so on.

Growing ginseng under natural hardwood shade makes use of idle land and eases the up-front investment.

Natural Shade

Ginseng will grow under any type of deciduous tree as long as the soil is good. The shade under pines is usually too heavy for ginseng growth, but a few pines, particularly white pines, scattered in a hardwood plot won't inhibit ginseng. In fact, I seek out white pines when I hunt wild ginseng because I often find some nice ginseng plants around the trees. I attribute the association of white pines and ginseng to birds that seek shelter in the pines and then deposit their droppings—which often contain ginseng seeds—in the vicinity. Always avoid areas that appear too dreary to hold any natural vegetation, unless you plan to do substantial pruning to allow some filtered sunlight into the area.

When selecting an area for a natural-shade garden, the first thing I do is walk around the woodlot checking for direct sunlight at various times during the day. Woodlands are naturally cooler than fields, so ginseng will tolerate some direct sunlight under trees. A good dappling effect is what I search for, with shadows shifting across the plot throughout the day. Direct sunlight for an hour or so in the early morning can be acceptable as long as those sections of the bed have a good high shade during the rest of the day. A filtered shade from the crowns of mature trees is perfect. I'm always aware, of course, that I might have to put up additional artificial shade if too much light leaks through in certain areas. Still, I look for areas with as much sunlight as ginseng can tolerate, since it experiences better root growth toward the high end of the acceptable light-intensity scale.

Keep in mind that some companion plants will tolerate sunlight better than ginseng, so only use good weeds as an indication of soil quality. Assess the shade separately.

When choosing natural shade, remember that the types of trees in your woodlot can affect your cultivation techniques. Equipment used for mounding beds and harvesting roots may be damaged by tree roots, and injuries inflicted on tree roots by equipment can kill trees, thereby reducing the shade cover. Shallow-rooted trees, such as maple, elm, and dogwood, are likely to give and receive more damage than more deeply rooted trees, such as oak, hickory, and beech.

All types of tree roots will rapidly invade your fertile ginseng beds. After all, trees are the rulers of the forest and seek out the most fertile soil for their own sustenance. Sacrificing some of your garden nutrients to produce healthy shade isn't all that big a deal, but the underground web of stringy tree roots becomes a nuisance during harvest.

Artificial Shade

The two types of artificial shade in wide use today for field-cultivated ginseng are wood-lathe shade and polypropylene fabric shade. Wood-lathe shade made from one-and-one-half-inch wide lathe strips tacked to twelve-foot runners was once the most popular type of shade with Wisconsin growers, but its use has fallen to about 50 percent in the last few years. Wood prices are up, and the panels can be difficult to handle and store over the winter.

Wood-lathe shade has some advantages over fabric shade for the backyard cultivator who has no natural shade but wants to raise some ginseng for personal use or as a side business. The materials for wood-lathe shade are easily obtained and can be built at home with a minimum of fuss. First I'll tell you how the professionals make and use wood-lathe shade; then I'll mention some shortcuts for the backyard cultivator.

Wood-lathe shade is constructed by stapling four-foot lengths of one-and-one-half-inch wide wood lathe to twelve-foot lengths of one-by-three lumber. Wood lathe is usually sold in bundles of fifty; lathe and one-by-three lumber are available at many lumber yards.

To construct a single panel, lay three one-by-three boards parallel to each other and on edge like runners on a sled. The outer runners are four feet apart; the middle runner is centered between them. Starting at one end, lay a single lathe strip across the one-by-threes and staple (or nail) it to each one-by-three. Lay another lathe strip one-half inch from the first, and staple it in place. To save time in measuring, use a one-half-inch dowel rod as your spacing guide; just hold it between the lathe strips while you staple them into place. Proceed in this fashion until you have completed a lathe shade panel. When finished, you'll see that placing one-and-one-half-inch strips one-half inch apart gives about 75 percent shade. Add in the shade offered by the three runners and you have approximately 78 percent, ideal for ginseng cultivation.

Now that you have one four-by-twelve-foot wood-lathe shade panel, how many more will you need? Only 899 if you intend to cover an acre!

On commercial ginseng farms, eight-foot or ten-foot posts are set one-and-one-half to two feet deep *in the raised beds.* The posts are generally set twelve feet apart. Heavy support beams or two-by-

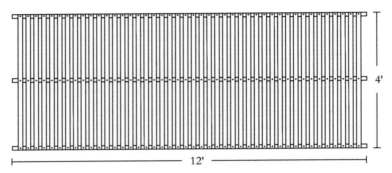

Twelve-foot wood-lathe shade panel

sixes are nailed to them to form a framework that the panels sit atop. This creates a "ceiling" across the garden. The overhead shade panels must extend beyond the border of the garden on the south, east, and west sides in order to avoid sunburn on the plants near the edge. These edge panels are often sloped downward to intercept more of the sunlight that can angle into the garden perimeter. After the growing season is over, the shade panels are removed and stacked for winter storage.

Since a six-foot-high wood-lathe structure may not be aesthetically pleasing in your backyard (a modest backyard garden tends to look a lot like an Indian burial edifice) and the thought of tossing around twelve-foot long panels may not appeal to you, a bit of tinkering with the commercial design might be in order to suit your needs.

A low-shade garden can be constructed with shade panels made from eight-foot sections of one-by-three runners with the support posts only three feet above the ground. The shorter panels are easier to handle, and the three-foot height is not nearly so obtrusive. If you want to reduce the weight of the panels even more, only two one-by-three runners need be used. In this case, nail the runners eight inches in from each edge.

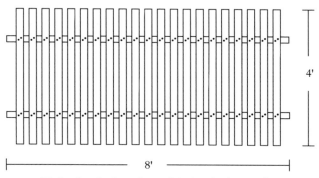

Eight-foot backyard wood-lathe shade panel

Although the low-shade design requires that you lift the panels to access the plants, the small garden can be hidden behind a dog kennel, a garage, or a shed. In fact, just a few shade panels in a lean-to design can suffice on the north side of a building, fence, or row of shrubbery. Korean growers use a thatched lean-to design for their shade, with bed direction thirty degrees from east to south and an open north face.

Fabric shade made from polypropylene cloth is growing in popularity with commercial growers because it requires little maintenance. It is destined to become the dominant shade for field-cultivated ginseng over the next few years. It is not often used by backyard growers since the fabric is sold in large rolls, and installation requires considerable expertise in stringing and tightening cable.

The polypropylene shade fabric is woven in a mixed opaque/translucent mesh providing 78 percent shade for ginseng. Its ultraviolet-blocking black color protects the fabric and maintains the proper shade by holding reflected light to a minimum. The porous weave allows rain to penetrate and permits some air circulation. The fabric is stretched over cables that are strung between posts in the raised beds.

Fabric comes in varying widths, but the most common is 24 feet. At this width, a section run of 168 feet is about the most two installers will be able to handle at one time.

The posts in a fabric shade "house" are generally set at twenty-four by twenty-four feet (or a slightly wider twenty-four feet, four inches to allow a good stretch in the fabric), although twelve-by-twenty-four-foot spacing is used if more cable support is required. The end post in each line of posts is anchored with a deadman anchor and wrap (a log buried lengthwise with a cable around the middle stretching to the top of the end post) in order to maintain the necessary tension on the cables. The interior posts are not anchored but are simply set in holes, although some growers do use tie-down cable anchors between posts.

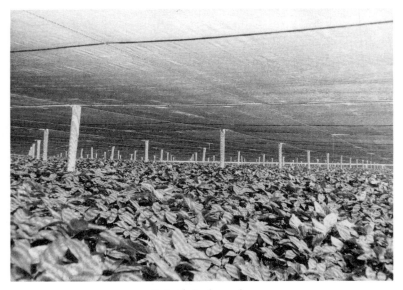

Fabric shade garden

A new grower might wonder why the interior garden posts are not moored, since the fabric covering is like a gigantic hang glider waiting to pull up roots and head off into the wild blue yonder during a good blow. That does happen, but not often. The fabric on a sizable garden weighs several tons, so it takes quite an updraft to get it rocking. When Mother Nature does roar, however, growers want to avoid two things: (1) tearing out all the grommets and cable connectors and (2) seeing a major part of their investment floating off into parts unknown. If disaster strikes and the fabric heads skyward, the interior posts don't stay in the ground but instead pop free and ride along underneath the billowing cloth. Since the posts act as weights, the whole mess usually crashes back to earth within a few hundred yards—grommets, cables, and posts intact. The grower then untangles the snarl and resets the shade before the exposed ginseng succumbs to sunburn.

One point of importance is the direction in which the fabric shade or lathe panels are placed. Either type of artificial shade should be erected so that the shade strips run in a north-south direction. This will allow an alternating dark/light pattern to fall across each plant in the garden as the sun moves from east to west. Shade strips that run in an east-west direction would let direct sunlight to fall on the same portion of the light-sensitive leaves throughout the day. Don't fret if your plot layout cannot accommodate a direct north-south position for the shade strips; simply get as close as you can.

Air circulation is vitally important for the health of the ginseng garden. The air under fabric shade is somewhat hotter than under wood-lathe shade due to heat generated by the black material and poorer air circulation, but as you move away from the six-foot-high shade toward soil level, thermal differences are minimal. Seed production and overall root growth are slightly lower under fabric shade, but ease in maintenance and storage make it the choice of the professionals.

Shade fabric for ginseng can be purchased from several dealers. Use of this type of shade also requires cable and connectors, so let the dealer know exactly what you have in mind when you talk to him or her about the purchase of shade fabric. The shade dealer will also be able to advise you on the basic design of a fabric shade garden. Most distributors will custom-fit their shade structures to your garden, so don't be afraid to ask questions when contacting fabric shade retailers. Addresses of shade dealers are listed in the Appendix.

PLOT ASSESSMENT

Once you have determined how you will provide the ginseng with the necessary shade, it's a good idea to assess the rest of your plot's characteristics. Proper drainage is a good starting point. Areas with standing water at any time of the year are out, as ginseng doesn't like to get its "feet" wet. Gentle to moderate slopes are ideal. North-facing slopes get the least direct sunlight and make for the coolest gardens. Northern slopes also hold the most wild ginseng, indicating a preference for that type of light, but wild ginseng grows on any slope as long as it gets proper shade. Gradients facing east, west, and south get correspondingly more direct sunlight and are therefore a bit warmer. The important thing to remember is to never plant at the bottom of a slope, because this is the area likely to be the wettest. Leave the low ground as a drainage area and plant higher on the slope, but check the soil carefully before planting at the crest of a hill. Reduced yields may be encountered on sandy ridge tops, since a garden there will be considerably drier than on side slopes.

Good soil grows good ginseng. Ginseng is naturally a denizen of light forest loam, preferring a loose, friable soil over a compacted clay soil. The quality of soil is important because it influences the taste, and therefore the value, of the roots. Organic matter approaching 4 percent in the upper layer is a real plus. In general, ginseng thrives in mellow, well-drained soil with a modest water-holding capacity in the top eight to twelve inches. Arid soils will stress the plants. Still, a little dry is better than a little wet. A dry, sandy soil can be amended with compost to enhance its water-retaining properties.

Studies have shown that the most important soil characteristic influencing ginseng growth is pH, or potential hydrogen. This is measured on a linear scale, with 7 being neutral. A pH of less than 7 is acid; greater than 7 is alkaline. Different plants require different pH ranges in order to efficiently use nutrients from the soil. In ginseng cultivation, the proper pH will influence root shape, size, and weight. Ginseng likes a slightly acidic soil, which is the normal condition of woodland soil under many deciduous trees. A pH below about 5.5 or above 6.5 can often curtail root growth. Most growers recognize a pH of 5.6 to 5.8 as ideal.

Soil pH can be altered through amendments to bring it into ginseng's preferred range. Problems with pH usually occur on the low, or acid, end of the scale, particularly under stands of oak, which can withstand a very sour soil. Lime, being alkaline, can be added to sour, or very acidic, soil. Lime adds crucial calcium and tends to enhance the uptake of phosphate by the ginseng plant. This results in greater root weight and a better shape. Raising the alkalinity, or sweetness, of the soil too far, however, can reduce resistance to disease. Usually, pH should not be raised above 6.0 with amendments.

If the soil is too sweet to grow ginseng successfully—a rare problem in woodland gardens—leaf and bark compost usually have a mild acidifying effect on soil and can often offer a slight correction. Aluminum sulfate and sulfur are also good soil acidifiers.

SOIL TESTING

It's a good idea to have your soil tested before adding any amendments. Ask your county extension agent for advice on where to pick up a soil sample kit: Usually a state university will run the test for a modest fee of under $10. Listing ginseng as your crop, ship the soil bag as indicated, and within a few weeks you'll receive a printout of your soil characteristics and recommendations for amendments, such as lime or fertilizer. You may have to wait a little longer than the time specified on the packet for the results because ginseng is considered a specialty crop and the sample is generally forwarded to a specialty agronomist for examination. The information you receive will be a very general guide, but it is a relatively inexpensive first step for your ginseng garden. If the results tell you that the site is unsuitable, you're out of the ginseng business at that location with very little invested. If you get a good report, follow the guidelines for any improvements and add amendments at least several months before planting.

Several private labs specialize in testing soil for ginseng. Their technicians can provide you with an extremely detailed analysis with recommendations for bringing your soil to maximum productivity for ginseng. They will also analyze plant tissue for the presence of disease and proper nutrient balance. These services can be expensive. One of these specialty labs is K Ag Laboratories International, Inc., operated by Dr. Akhtar Khwaja. Dr. Khwaja is quite experienced in ginseng analysis, and he recommends four samples per plot be tested, starting with a soil analysis in the fall. In his schedule, another soil analysis is done in the spring and plant tissue specimens are taken in June and August. Expect to pay at least $250 per site for these services.

Another method of soil analysis that has been used by some diggers and growers is to simply follow what nature does best. They take soil samples from around large wild ginseng plants and then bring their woodland garden soil to that level of fertility. Others have learned to recognize the best ginseng soil through years of digging wild ginseng. Still others are able to identify companion plants and simply sow ginseng seeds near them. Unless you are particularly adept in these endeavors, however, a laboratory analysis of your ginseng plot soil is a wise investment.

SOIL PREPARATION

The soil for a ginseng garden should be worked several times in the year preceding planting to bring weed seeds to the surface, where they sprout and are cut off in subsequent tillings. For field-cultivated ginseng, plows and disks are used. Similar equipment can be used in a forest setting, although mobility is somewhat limited by the trees.

Many small-plot cultivators use a garden tiller under natural shade with good results. Brush and large leaf litter must be moved aside before tilling in the woods. Decayed humus can be left to be worked into the soil. Rear-tine tillers work better in woodland gardens because they tend to jump less than front-tine tillers when roots are hit—which will happen often. The leaf litter that has been gathered can be shredded and tilled into the plot on a subsequent tilling as a compost.

Soil amendments are also worked into the ground during these tillings. If you have a fertilizer recommendation as a result of a soil test, follow the guidelines. I like to add bone meal as an organic fertilizer on the last tilling before planting. Bone meal contains phosphorus and calcium, both of which are critical to good root development in ginseng. It is vitally important to work phosphate amendments six to eight inches into the soil during tilling. Phosphorus tends to stay where it is placed, so now is the time to get it down where the roots can use it.

The Koreans, known for their painstaking approach to ginseng cultivation, prepare soil in one of three methods, depending upon soil types and organic material to be added. The most popular method, called Yang-Jig, is also the most expensive, but it is considered well worth the cost and effort because of the quality of root it produces. The formula is quite interesting and may offer some guidance to the American cultivator.

In Yang-Jig, the field is plowed fifteen times in the summer before planting, mixing the green leaves of small bushes into the soil. When the soil is mellow, beds are prepared by adding eighteen parts virgin granite soil, two parts sand, and nine parts Yakto (a mix of completely composted leaves, soybean cakes, and bone meal).

Woodland gardens can be laid out much like field-cultivated plots, planting in rows through the shade structures, which, in this case, are living trees. Anything that may damage tree roots should be used with caution. When preparing a tract, I like to use a heavy duty mower like a brush hog to clear the low brush, then disk

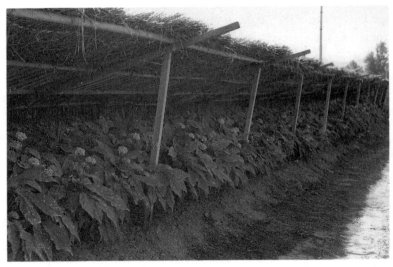

Korean ginseng garden (photo courtesy of Hsu's Ginseng Enterprises)

lightly to about six inches in June. I find that the chopped vegetation adds some organic material to the soil. A layer of two inches of compost can also be worked in nicely with a disk if additional organic material is required.

I don't mound the soil on slopes. Ginseng doesn't grow in mounded soil naturally, and if you've picked a suitable site, it's unnecessary work. Sites that are a little low or poorly drained, however, will definitely benefit from mounding.

After disking, I let the area sit for about a month, during which I may put out some slug pellets around the perimeter if a light rain is forecast. Slug pellets work best when they're moist but not wet, and I take advantage of a damp, muggy evening to thin out the slug population. Sometime in August I'll spray the disked area and perimeter with a herbicide to knock down any weeds that sprouted after the soil was turned. Mayapples, poison ivy, and Virginia creeper should be attacked with a vengeance, since they will overrun your garden in a few short years if they become established. If you start this a year before you plan to plant you'll have a much cleaner garden (some of the weeds are very tenacious), but I never seem to find the time to spend two summers preparing a ginseng garden.

PLANTING BEDS

For field-cultivated and woodsgrown ginseng, raised planting beds from four to six feet wide are formed where soil drainage may be a problem. The beds are built extending downhill—no contour farming here—so that excess water is pulled away from the ginseng roots as quickly as possible. These beds are crowned in the middle and slope off to paths, or trenches, on each side. The beds may be raised anywhere from a few inches to a few feet above the paths. The crown height is determined by the slope of the land. Steeper slopes require less elevation in the bed because water moves away quickly.

Standard beds in Wisconsin commercial gardens are four and

a half feet wide with one-and-a-half-foot trenches on each side. The trenches are actually the tracks for the equipment used in the gardens. Professional growers find that this size bed is easy to work with in weeding and spray applications. This layout is also compatible with twelve- or twenty-four-foot midbed post spacing (4½-foot bed + two 1½-foot trenches + two 2¼-foot half-beds = 12-foot or doubled, 24-foot).

Beds can be constructed in several ways. When using a shovel, soil from the trenches is shoveled up onto the beds. A suitable bed can also be formed with a tractor and plow by cutting furrows where the trenches will be. Commercial ginseng growers use custom bed-makers.

Growers planning artificial-shade cultivation may want to fumigate the beds before planting. This entails applying a fumigant to the soil after it is worked and then covering it with plastic for ten days. Fumigants are nonselective poisons that have the potential to kill any living thing. Commonly employed in tobacco beds, they destroy fungal spores, roots, seeds, insects, and nematodes. Methyl bromide was at one time the most commonly used fumigant, but it is being phased out over the next five to ten years because of concerns about bromide buildup in the soil. Vorlex is another fumigant that is being discontinued by the manufacturer. The two replacement fumigants are Vapam and Basamid. Vapam is water-soluble and is applied as a liquid. Basamid is granular and is applied as a top dressing on the soil surface.

Fumigants have a low vapor pressure, so they change to gas as they enter the soil and permeate every square inch of the bed. A plastic covering is required to hold the toxic gas in the soil. Commercial applicators use small injectors to place the chemical into the soil, but good results can be obtained by sprinkling with a common sprinkling can. After removing the plastic, the bed should be aerated for about six weeks before planting ginseng seeds or roots. Fumigants cannot be used in natural shade gardens because they may kill the trees.

SEEDS AND ROOTLETS

Ginseng beds are usually planted with stratified seed or rootlets, although green seeds are sometimes sown in woodland gardens. Stratified seeds have been held in moist sand for one year and are offered for sale the autumn after they were picked. These seeds will sprout the next spring. Green seeds are freshly picked kernels that have not yet been stratified. Green seed is cheaper and can be planted under natural shade but you will have to wait an extra year to see your ginseng plants sprout. Green seed is never planted under artificial shade, due to the cost of setting up and maintaining shade over dormant seeds. Don't confuse green seed with green

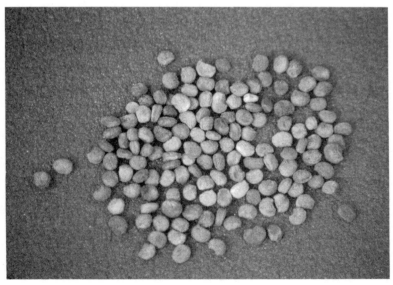

Ginseng seeds

berries, as some novice growers have done. Green berries are unripe and should not be picked until they turn red.

Stratified seed can be purchased from large ginseng operations, several of which advertise in outdoor magazines each fall. It is important to buy seeds from a dealer who water tests, or "floats," the seeds before stratifying. Floating simply entails dumping freshly picked and depulped seeds into a tub of water and skimming off the seeds that float to the surface. Floating seeds are not fully formed and contain air within the shell, therefore are unable to produce a plant. Up to 20 percent of the seeds produced from any one plot can be expected to be bad. Since you won't want to take a 20 percent loss on your investment outright, deal only with a reputable grower for seed.

Northern seeds are larger and heavier than southern seeds. Expect to receive 6,000 to 7,500 seeds per pound for northern seed and up to 8,500 seeds per pound for southern seed. Both northern and southern seed are suitable for starting ginseng gardens just about anywhere in the plant's natural range, but to get the best possible yield, purchase seed from your own geographic region or one that has climatic conditions similar to your planting site.

Good-quality seed will have a germination rate of about 90 percent. Some gardeners report success rates of over 90 percent, while others report dismal germination rates as low as 50 percent. The lower rates almost always result from improper seeding or mulching, or severe predation by snails, slugs, chipmunks and mice, rather than from bad seeds. Remember, the professional grower will be planting his garden from the same seed stock as you, so the seeds are nearly always viable.

To tell if seeds are good, look them over carefully when you receive them. They should range from off-white to dark brown in color and be firm. Some of the seeds will have started to crack open by fall, and a bit of tiny white tendril may show along the side. This is normal and indicates a healthy seed. Seeds that are mushy or pulpy are not viable, and the condition of the shipment should be reported immediately to the seller. A reputable dealer will likely send another batch out immediately, but don't expect a dealer to replace seed that you have handled improperly.

Upon arrival, seeds should be opened and aired for several minutes—*but not dried*—before storing or planting. Seeds that are not to be planted promptly can be mixed with an equal amount of moist sand and placed in a cool place. A refrigerator or cool cellar can be used, but don't store the seeds in a freezer. If the seeds are to be held for an extended time, it's a good idea to check on them occasionally, stirring the sand and making sure it is still moist. Seeds that dry out will die.

Many gardeners treat their purchased seeds with captan, maneb, or a bleach solution to inhibit the transfer of diseases from commercial gardens. Captan stops hitchhiking fungal spores from attacking seedlings when they sprout. Bleach kills any spores attached to the seeds. Maneb tends to both kill spores and inhibit their ability to attack seedlings. While some growers believe treatment lowers the germination rate, weak solutions are probably a safe bet.

The mix ratio for captan or maneb seed treatment is one or two tablespoons of chemical agent to one gallon of water. Seeds are soaked in this mixture for about five minutes. I use maneb; captan has not been particularly effective in tests. An alternate method is to soak seeds for three to five minutes in a solution of one or two tablespoons of bleach to one gallon of water. Any of these treatments is also suitable for planting rootlets.

Rootlets, immature roots from one to three years old, can also be purchased for planting. They are more expensive than seeds and more time-consuming to plant but give a relatively quick return in seed production. A word of caution: planting rootlets is not a cost-effective method of starting ginseng for root sales. Rather, they are planted to jump-start seed production, since starting from seed requires at least a four-year wait for viable seeds from those plants. Using rootlets cuts that time in half. Therefore, new growers should consider reserving at least part of the plot for three-year-old, seed-producing rootlets. Starting a nice plot of well-spaced seed bearers will dramatically cut your seed costs for future plantings. Seed production varies widely for ginseng plants, but expect an average of thirty to forty viable seeds from each five-year-old plant. Younger plants obviously can be expected to produce less and older plants, more.

After you decide how many plants you will need to sustain your own seed requirements for future plantings, add about 5 percent for unavoidable losses. If the cost of these rootlets is prohibitive in the first year, spread out the purchase over two or more years. If you're going to be in the ginseng business, you're going to have to plan for seed production right from the start.

Wild roots, legally harvested, can be transplanted into a garden, although I do not encourage this practice. Wild plants often do poorly in the confines of a garden because they are more susceptible to disease than cultivated plants. Also, wild ginseng is becoming scarce in many areas. Depleting the natural population by transplanting wild roots to a garden is foolhardy in the long run. A few wild plants scattered around the seed-producing plot might be worthwhile for cross-pollination purposes, but I recommend that wild plants be left in the wild.

PLANTING

Ginseng seeds can be hand-cast and raked into the top layer of soil, scattered without raking and covered with mulch, or planted in rows with a mechanical device.

Broadcast sowing is quite acceptable in woodsgrown plantings. Seeds that are raked in to about one-half to three-quarter inch beneath the surface will experience less predation from rodents and slugs than seeds simply left on the top of the ground and covered with mulch. Seeds should not be planted deeper than one inch. The seeds must have some type of covering to maintain moisture, and nature conveniently provides it with a covering of fresh deciduous leaves each fall. For woodland growers, this might be the only mulch needed.

Seeds can also be planted with a garden planter that drops a single seed through a hole at a set spacing. Some tinkering with the seed plates may be required to get the results you desire. Small holes can be drilled out just enough for a single ginseng seed to drop through each opening. On large operations, mechanized seed drills pulled behind a tractor can be used, but expect some difficulty maneuvering the equipment in a forest.

The seeding rate varies widely. One hundred or more pounds per acre are planted under artificial shade. (One hundred pounds per acre ≈ 1.2-inch seed spacing in 6-inch rows.) This really packs the plants together at maturity and requires constant spraying to alleviate disease problems. As little as ten pounds per acre can be sown in woodsgrown cultivation. For a wild-simulated garden, you can simply walk through the woodland and plant seeds here and there in rich, fertile soil, or plant small, widely scattered patches of thirty or so seeds.

Spacing has a very definite effect on root growth in ginseng plants. The closer the spacing, the smaller the roots at harvest. Tight spacing increases the number of roots per acre, however, and therefore actually increases the total yield per acre as measured in gross weight. Artificial-shade growers are concerned only with the total weight since the roots are low quality anyway, and they have a tremendous investment in shade materials. Therefore, they grow as many plants per acre as possible. Woodland growers, on the other hand, tend to use wider spacing and produce fewer roots but receive a premium price for their efforts.

Studies have shown that under natural shade conditions a middle-of-the-road approach is most efficient in the ratio of harvest weight to seed investment. Here's why. Tight spacing of perhaps two by two inches on average requires a massive investment in seed just to cover the area. Many more roots will be produced on this plot than on a plot with an average spacing of six by nine inches. But the tightly spaced roots will tend to be spindly, whereas the well-spaced roots will be much larger and heavier due to reduced competition for available nutrients. This enhanced root growth is cumulative over the years. In an eight-year garden it is likely that the increased mass of the chunky, widely spaced roots will approach 75 percent of the total weight per acre of the more numerous but spindly, tightly spaced roots. And the larger roots will fetch a higher price per pound. With a greatly reduced seed investment and lower costs in chemical applications and labor (especially at harvest), wide spacing is often preferred under natural shade. Widely spaced ginseng plants also produce more berries per plant. The bottom line is that wide spacing between plants reduces the chances for disease, produces bigger and more valuable roots, and requires less work by the cultivator.

What is the best spacing for woodsgrown ginseng? Many growers use a six-by-six-inch spacing. Rootlets or seeds are planted every six inches in rows six inches apart. Even wider spacing can be used to cut down on the risk of disease transmission. Plants that do not touch each other are at less risk for disease and enjoy better overall development than plants that grow very close together. Some growers plant seedbeds with spacing of only one inch apart in six-inch rows and then transplant the roots to wider spacing after a year or two. Transplanting can give the roots a boost by loosening the soil, but it is labor intensive and exposes the ginseng to fungal diseases that may be unearthed during transplanting.

Although ginseng beds have traditionally been sown in the fall, year-old stratified ginseng seeds can be held until spring if they are buried or kept refrigerated, but they seem to have a built-in clock and begin to germinate in late April under all but the harshest conditions. They will start to sprout at about thirty-six degrees Fahrenheit. If wet weather keeps you out of your garden in the spring, the seeds may sprout before they can be planted, in which case they are lost. If only a small portion of the tendril is exposed, the seeds can still be successfully planted but should not be held longer than necessary. Spring planting lowers the exposure of seeds to pests, however, and some growers are experimenting with spring planting of seeds.

Planting or transplanting roots requires that each root be handled individually. This can be done only during a dormancy period or after the next year's bud has formed on the neck. Any plant attached to the root will wilt and die during transplanting.

The root is laid at an angle in a trench so the bud will be about one or two inches underground after the trench is covered. The other end of the root should face downward at an angle without cramping the tendrils. Cramping the fine tendrils can cause the end of the root to turn upward into a J or fishhook shape—a sure tip-off to an experienced buyer that a root has been transplanted. Many fishhook roots can lower your lot price, particularly if you are peddling your ginseng as wild or wild-simulated.

Roots that are very long and thin can be trimmed back to two to three inches to encourage a stockier root. A new, stubbier rootstock will sprout from the trimmed end. Trimming can allow disease to penetrate the root, so there is a risk.

Planting or transplanting roots should be considered a permanent endeavor. I don't recommend transplanting ginseng more than once during the life of the plant unless absolutely necessary. Make sure you have your spacing figured out in advance, and don't let the fine hair roots become dry. Cover and water the roots quickly in order to reduce shock.

FERTILIZATION

Ginseng, being a dwarf in a forest of giants, is used to getting by on slim pickings. If it sends its tiny tendrils out into the right direction, it may find a morsel of nourishment here or there that has just been laid down by the microorganisms in the woodland leaf mold, or it may chance upon a bit of phosphorus that has been bound up in a grain of soil since time immemorial, missed over the aeons by the invasive web of maple and hickory roots that ply every square inch of soil to feed their massive frames. Ginseng doesn't need much in the way of soil nutrients to survive or, in fact, flourish. Just about any moderately fertile soil is capable of supporting ginseng.

Whether to fertilize ginseng has been debated since the early days of American cultivation circa 1890. A century later there is still no definitive answer. Growers face two problems in fertilizing ginseng. Fertilizer tends to make ginseng more susceptible to disease, and quick growth brought on by fertilization results in a poorly ringed root. Purists argue that fertilization is a waste of money because ginseng naturally grows slowly. Fertilization does make for heavier roots, however. Both sides of the argument have avid followers, and you can decide whether to fertilize based on your personal preference for quality in the roots you produce. I think an occasional application of a light fertilizer is beneficial to the overall health of a ginseng garden.

Nitrogen, phosphorus, and potassium are the "big three" ginseng nutrients. You'll see them listed on any fertilizer bag by their percentage of total weight.

Nitrogen is responsible for top growth. It's the stuff that makes plants green and tall. It's also the stuff that microorganisms use in breaking down leaf mold. Since soil microbes use much of the available nitrogen in a forest setting, ginseng is used to doing without much of it.

Phosphorus is listed next, and it's good for the bottom end: the root. It also enhances seed production. Phosphorus doesn't move much in the soil but tends to stay within a couple of inches of where it has been placed by man or nature. Therefore, banding phosphate several inches deep is critical for maximum root growth.

Potassium brings up the tail end of the label, and it's good for everything between the root and the leaves. Potassium gives overall strength and good disease resistance to plants.

A host of micronutrients critical for any plant's survival are found naturally in most soils. These are a little more troublesome to compensate for if one or more is greatly lacking. Calcium is one micronutrient that is critical for ginseng growth. It is a natural component of lime and bone meal and is included in some commercial fertilizer blends.

Organic soil amendments are topnotch for supplementing micronutrients as well as macronutrients if you intend to add fertilizers. Leaf mold and compost are good additions and add much-needed organic material to the soil. Either chemical or organic fertilizers may be used for ginseng, but organic fertilizers usually contain a number of natural micronutrients that can aid in growth and disease resistance.

Fertilizers can affect the flavor of ginseng roots. Early growers discovered that fresh manure was not a good fertilizer for ginseng when Asian buyers complained that the roots tasted like animal dung. Manure is now used only if mixed with compost materials and aged for a year before application. Chemical fertilizers can also give roots a chemical "bite."

Growers using commercial fertilizers generally depend on a light application of a standard 10-10-10 or 15-30-15 blend, while organic growers rely simply upon compost or an organic-based fertilizer. Many growers give their seedling beds a shot of nitrogen fertilizer early in the season to compensate for the nitrogen being used by microorganisms in breaking down the new mulch. Korean ginseng farmers are partial to leaf mulch, pulverized granite, and bone meal as supplements.

Foliar feeding is gaining widespread acceptance in the ginseng industry. Foliar fertilizers are mixed with water and sprayed onto the plant's foliage, where the nutrients are absorbed directly through the leaves. Again, either chemical or organic compounds can be used in this method. Foliar fertilizers can be combined with a fungicide drench to feed and protect the plants in a single application.

In forest gardens, withholding fertilization during the last two growing seasons can improve the quality of the roots by slowing their growth. Slow growth encourages the roots to develop wrinkles, or rings, which greatly increase their value.

MULCH

Ginseng seeds germinate under a blanket of leaves in their natural forest setting; therefore, a mulch covering on the ginseng garden is considered essential by most growers. Mulch protects newly sown ginseng seeds from drying out and reflects heat from the soil, lowering soil temperatures to ginseng's liking. It also helps insulate the ginseng beds from freeze-thaw cycles during the winter.

A number of different mulches have been used for ginseng, but chopped straw is the most popular among commercial growers. Oat straw is considered the best because it contains few seeds, and those that might find their way to the garden often sprout in the fall and are killed by the frost. Wheat straw is also used; any sprouts that appear are killed by a herbicide before the ginseng plants appear in the spring. Pure, fine-chip sawdust is generally avoided because it cakes, and plants have a hard time breaking through the crust. Also, many farmers believe fine-chip sawdust harbors fungal diseases that attack seedlings. Other mulches, such as pine needles, large-chip sawdust, chipped bark, and hardwood leaves, have been tried with varying levels of success. Interestingly, the type of mulch you use may influence the weight gain in your roots.

A study by Tom Konsler of the North Carolina Extension Service presented at the second annual ginseng conference showed that an oak sawdust and bark mulch gave the best overall root weight gain in one of his test plots. Its performance was followed by poplar sawdust and bark, pine sawdust and bark, hardwood leaves, straw, and pine needles, in that order. Interestingly, the natural mulch of hardwood leaves did not give the best results in this particular study. The commercial growers' choice, straw, was ranked even lower. Many factors can influence growth rates under any mulch, however, including soil characteristics, degree of mulch decomposition, microbial activity, temperature, moisture, and even the age of the plants. Therefore, results often vary in commercial practice. Still, if different mulches are available in your area, it might be wise to experiment on various tracts to see what type of mulch works best for you.

Straw can be blown or hand-scattered over the beds to a depth of three to four inches. This will pack down to about one and a half inches over the winter. That's about as much mulch as you'll want, particularly on seedbeds. Seedlings can have a tough time pushing up through a heavy mulch.

Leaves from deciduous trees are often the mulch of choice in woodland gardens. Tough leaves, such as oak, are hard for seedlings to push through. They can be shredded or chopped before spreading. A number of commercial leaf shredders are available, and some small-plot growers mince leaves by running over them several times with a lawn mower.

CARING FOR PLANTS

Intensively cultivated ginseng gardens require much care. Professional growers either work at it full time or hire a farm manager to handle all the chores.

Before your plants come up, you should check the mulch. Add to areas that have been swept clean by the winter winds and thin a little from areas where it is piled up. A spray of weed control can be used early if you detect a great number of weeds sprouting, but this should be done with extreme caution. Any ginseng plants that have poked through the mulch will be killed by the spray along with the weeds.

Artificial shade is generally erected before the ginseng plants

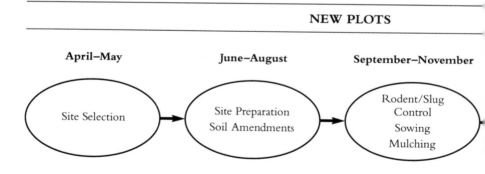

NEW PLOTS

April–May	June–August	September–November
Site Selection	Site Preparation Soil Amendments	Rodent/Slug Control Sowing Mulching

Flow chart of ginseng cultivation

come up. During wet springs, the shade can be delayed until most of the plants are showing to prevent fungal diseases from forming. Seedbeds are particularly susceptible to early damp-weather diseases. Korean growers usually wait until 30 percent of their seedlings emerge before putting up shade. Erecting shade after the plants have sprouted requires a little more caution to avoid trampling the plants, but heading off fungal disease is usually worth the extra effort.

Older plants sprout earlier than the new seedlings. There is about a five-day delay for each year class down from the mature plants; that is, two-year-old plants will sprout about five days later than three- and four-year-olds, and seedlings will sprout about five to seven days later than the two-year-olds. So put shade on the older beds first.

The emergence date for ginseng varies widely with the cli-

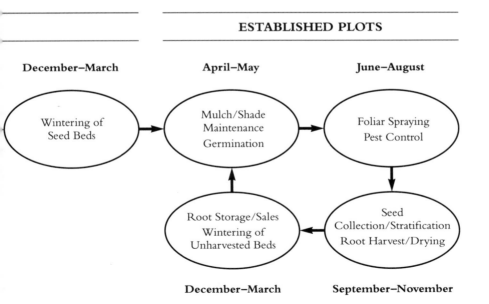

ESTABLISHED PLOTS

December–March　　　　**April–May**　　　　**June–August**

Wintering of Seed Beds → Mulch/Shade Maintenance Germination → Foliar Spraying Pest Control

Root Storage/Sales Wintering of Unharvested Beds ← Seed Collection/Stratification Root Harvest/Drying

December–March　　　　**September–November**

mate. The bowed heads of the mature plants begin showing in southern zone 6 by the third week of April. In colder zones, they may not show for another three weeks. Expect a total emergence period of up to three weeks. Plants respond differently to stimuli, and some hold back a little, perhaps as an instinct to avoid frost damage. The earlier plants get a few extra days of growth and a crack at finding the best sunlight, but they also risk frost damage.

Weeds will also sprout in your fertile garden soil. Weeding is a very labor-intensive task in ginseng cultivation. Most artificial-shade growers weed their gardens to reduce competition for nutrients. Woodland growers are divided on the necessity of weeding, since pulling weeds can bring disease spores to the surface. A few weeds in the woodland ginseng garden do not pose a real problem, and some cultivators believe that weeds actually reduce the incidence of disease by their diversity. Weeds that threaten to overtake the garden should be dealt with. They can be pulled, or cut off above the ginseng's level with a weed-trimming machine. A few growers "wick" the weeds when they grow higher than the ginseng plants. This entails drawing a treated wand across the beds above the ginseng. A herbicide in the wand rubs off as it crosses the weeds and kills them within a few days.

Chapter 5

Ginseng Diseases and Pests

In one word, it [ginseng] will make a man live a great while, and very well while he does live . . . however 'tis of little use in the feats of love, as a great prince once found, who hearing of its invigorating quality, sent as far as China for some of it, though his ladys could not boast of any advantage thereby.

William Byrd,
Virginia planter and satirist,
circa 1729

D isease and pest control starts soon after the ginseng plants emerge under intensive cultivation. It is the practice of many growers to use both a fungicide such as maneb and an insecticide, such as diazinon, for control. These are generally delivered as a foliar spray, but dusting—sprinkling the plants with a very fine coating— is also effective. Sprays can be delivered by machine-mounted mechanical sprayers in commercial operations or by backpack sprayers in smaller woodland gardens.

DISEASES

Fungal diseases are common on cultivated ginseng and are spread by wind, water, or direct contact between healthy and diseased plants. Spores can also be carried on clothing and tools. Crowded conditions in a garden promote disease for several reasons. Close contact and high humidity make it easier for the spores to spread, which increases the likelihood of fungal contamination. Spores can overwinter in dead plants and mulch and are ready to attack when conditions become favorable the next spring. Fungus diseases are most likely to appear during wet or humid weather, when their hyphae are stimulated to penetrate healthy plant tissue.

Alternaria

Alternaria panax is the most common stem and leaf blight of culti- vated ginseng. It is not believed to specifically infect other agricul- ture crops but is closely related to *Alternaria solani,* a disease of tomatoes. I suspect some native woodland flora may harbor Alter- naria because the infection is occasionally found on wild ginseng plants. The fungal disease will attack all parts of the plant but is usually found on the stems, leaves, and flower peduncle.

Airborne spores of Alternaria are blown from infected plants to unaffected garden plots, where they lodge on healthy plants and germinate when a film of water or dew is present on the plant. Stimulated by moisture, the spores send tiny, threadlike mycelia into the plant cells, causing the fungal disease. During humid weather, the fungus produces chains of spores and releases them into the air, repeating the cycle as the newly formed spores fall on healthy plants.

The first symptoms of Alternaria are generally lesions on the stem or leaf. Stem cankers are brown and up to two inches in length. They become darker and velvety as spores are produced and can enlarge to encircle the stem. Nutrient uptake is diminished or stopped, and the plant often bends and falls over. Infections of the seed stalks are similar and will cause the flower or berries to drop off.

Leaf cankers are often circular or wedge shaped. In humid weather, the lesions are a soggy green color; during dry weather they turn brown and papery, eventually dropping away to leave a hole in the leaf. The lesions are often surrounded by a yellow margin, helping distinguish Alternaria leaf blight from Phytophthora leaf blight.

Root infection can occur, causing a dark rot, but this is not very common. It occurs only if the blight works its way down the stem and into the root. Bud infections from stem blight can result in the loss of the next year's bud, setting the plant back a full year in growth.

Alternaria can start anywhere in a garden and spreads rapidly if left unchecked. It is generally more severe in artificial-shade gardens, where temperature and humidity tend to be slightly higher than under natural shade.

Alternaria spores overwinter in mulch and infected ginseng debris. These spores infect ginseng stalks as they break through the mulch each spring, causing early-season stem blight and setting the stage for large numbers of spores to be produced.

The primary method of spore dispersal is wind, but spores can be carried on clothing, tools and animal fur.

There is no way to cure an Alternaria outbreak; the grower

must simply strive to prevent and control the disease. Sanitation in gardens is a major step in disease prevention. Some small-plot cultivators pick up all the debris and mulch off their gardens each year in order to remove the spores that may have settled there. The infected mulch is then buried or disposed of. Infected plants can also be cut off at ground level and removed from the garden (the root will send up another plant the following year if the disease has not infected the bud). Running a bagging mower over a garden is a handy way to pick up loose mulch and ginseng debris on smaller plots.

Cultivators should not walk from infected gardens into uninfected plots without changing clothing and shoes. A safe practice is to tend your infected plots last, so as not to unintentionally carry spores to your healthy plants. Animals used for rodent control (ferrets or cats) should not be permitted to roam between diseased and healthy garden beds. The same holds true for guard dogs fenced inside gardens. Since airborne Alternaria spores are abundant, however, these steps are likely only to reduce incidence of disease, not stop it completely.

Disease control is effected through the use of fungicides such as maneb, captan, Aliette, and Benlate. Fungicide combinations are often used by commercial growers to get the widest possible range of protection. Spreader-stickers are generally used, and good coverage is essential. Alternaria control entails spraying every ten to fourteen days during the growing season and after frequent leaf wettings.

Phytophthora

Phytophthora cactorium is a soilborne fungus that produces two infections in ginseng, a leaf blight and a root rot. The leaf blight is not as common as Alternaria but may resemble Alternaria somewhat in appearance. Unlike the airborne spores of Alternaria, Phytophthora is carried by water.

Phytophthora leaf blight is characterized by lesions that appear as dark green, watery wilted areas on the leaf. Later the lesions become brown, papery, and then nearly transparent. Phytophthora leaf blight can also resemble heat and drought injury, as well as Alternaria.

Heavy rain and cool temperatures can spark a Phytophthora outbreak through spores splashing onto the foliage. Spores can also hitch a ride on infected clothing and equipment, so stay out of your gardens while the plants are wet. Phytophthora needs several hours of wet conditions in order to develop. Infected plants spread the disease quickly through contact with healthy leaves.

Phytophthora root rot is similar to the blight on potatoes, *Phytophthora infestans,* that caused the great potato famine in Ireland many years ago. It spreads rapidly in older gardens, reducing root quality and killing the plants. Since it is carried with water, the disease often moves downhill along the contour of a garden. The disease is so virulent that entire gardens can be destroyed in a few weeks.

Wilting plants are usually the first indication of a Phytophthora root infection. Affected roots are rubbery and off-white in color. As the disease progresses, liquid can be squeezed from the root and a foul odor can be detected. Late-season infection in mature gardens may go unnoticed until the roots are harvested and dried. Dark discoloration in dried roots is indicative of a Phytophthora infection and reduces the market value of the product.

Phytophthora produces several types of spores. Zoospores are one-celled spores that actually swim through a film of water to attack a ginseng root or leaf. They form cysts that germinate and develop mycelium inside the plant tissue, causing it to rot. Thick-walled oospores capable of overwintering in soil are then formed inside the root, causing further damage. In the spring, oospores germinate and eventually produce the mobile zoospores that spread the disease. Oospores can survive for many years and are capable of infecting other plant species. Beds infected with Phytophthora cannot be used again.

Sanitation is a must in controlling Phytophthora. Any equipment used in diseased beds should be thoroughly hosed down and allowed to dry before moving it to healthy beds. Hand tools and boots can be rinsed with a one-to-ten bleach/water solution.

Diseased plants should be removed from a garden, roots and all. Healthy plants within eighteen inches of the diseased plants should also be removed. Most growers recommend destroying these healthy "perimeter" plants as a precaution, but you may want to soak the roots in fungicide solution for a few minutes and replant them some distance from your garden. Those that have not been infected will sprout disease free the following year.

Systemic fungicides such as Ridomil, Aliette, and Benlate are effective when used as part of a continuing spray program but may contaminate roots with chemical residue if used too close to harvest. Leaf and stem blight fungicides can be used as foliar protectants to keep the spores from germinating on the leaves.

Avoidance is the best way to reduce the risk of Phytophthora infections. Poor drainage contributes to the conditions favored by this fungus. Raised beds with high levels of organic material can control Phytophthora through good soil drainage and microorganisms that naturally inhibit the fungus.

Rust

Rust and rusty root describe two different diseases that cause redbrown rust spots to appear on ginseng roots. Fusarium and Cylindrocarpon fungi are always found in association with rust disease on ginseng but do not seem to cause the disease by themselves. Infected plants may simply fail to appear in the spring or may turn yellow and wilt. The roots can disintegrate, but many times they will heal themselves, leaving behind a scar. Alkaline soils seem to be favored by the fungi that cause the rust diseases.

It is likely that a number of biological factors combine to form the rust on ginseng. Because research is incomplete, no controls are known. Certain soil bacteria naturally suppress fungi, and these may protect wild ginseng. A relatively low soil pH may reduce the impact of rust and rusty root. Fungicides for foliar rust on wheat are not effective on ginseng root rust. Research for development of an effective rust control on ginseng is under way.

Black Root Rot

Black root rot is caused by the fungus *Stromatinia panacis* (formerly called *Sclerotinia panacis*), which occurs naturally in the forest soil. It is a rare disease of ginseng that makes the root look mummified with a black skin. The inside of the root becomes white and watery. Stromatinia is also responsible for white rot, a variation that causes the rotting portion of the root to turn white instead of black. This fungus grows best in cool weather and rarely appears during the summer months. When seen, it is usually during fall or spring.

Black root rot is a rarity and is not thought of as a threat to ginseng cultivation. Infected roots cannot be saved. The root and surrounding soil should be removed and destroyed when discovered. Copper sulfate can be used to disinfect the beds.

Damping Off and Tip-Over

Ginseng seedlings are quite vulnerable to soilborne fungi during the first few weeks of growth. Attacks by root pathogens cause the plant to collapse at soil level, or "damp-off." Fungi that attack the stem above the soil level cause "tip-over" when a lesion weakens the stem and it falls over. Damping-off is caused by at least four fungi, of which pythium is the most common. Tip-over is caused by the fungus *Rhizoctonia solani*. Wet, cool weather at the beginning of the growing season contributes to the spread of these diseases.

A light mulch is preventative in controlling both diseases. Heavy mulches harbor pathogens and slow ginseng's emergence. Dense sawdust mulch can contribute to damping-off, since it retains moisture and crusts. Cool weather hastens the diseases, so some growers wait until seedling plants have emerged to cover them with shade. This allows the ground to warm faster and reduces damping-off. Other growers saturate their beds with maneb just as the plants emerge in the spring.

Botrytis

Botrytis blight, caused by the fungus *Botrytis cinerea,* is a relatively uncommon pathogen on ginseng in the United States. It is much more common in Ontario. This is the same fungus that causes a gray mold on strawberries, raspberries, and grapes. It tends to be an opportunistic pathogen and often attacks through wounds on the plants. It can also use fallen petals on a leaf to set up shop and subsequently infect healthy plant tissue.

Botrytis is often first observed as a water-soaked lesion on the foliage. Spores, or conidia, soon arise from the surface of the infected tissue. This gray-white fuzz is dispersed into the air and then carried to healthy plants. Ginseng flowers and berries can also be infected with Botrytis. Infected red berries often become covered in a dense gray fuzz. Stem infections may cause wilted plants, like Phytophthora infections, but the roots of plants infected with Botrytis do not rot.

Good management practices are critical in reducing the incidence of Botrytis. Crowded conditions and poor ventilation create pockets of still, humid air that favor the disease. Mechanical damage from machinery can also invite Botrytis into your ginseng garden. There are currently no fungicides registered for control of Botrytis on ginseng, but fungicides labeled for Alternaria tend to suppress Botrytis to some extent.

INJURIES

Injuries to ginseng plants can come from two sources, the environment and chemicals.

Environmental Injury

Frost, heat, and drought can damage ginseng plants in ways similar to some diseases. Frost damage can result in twisted, misshapen plants, but plants hurt by frost usually survive with no ill effect to the root.

Heat and drought injury may mimic a fungal disease. Ginseng plants can become stressed during hot, dry weather and exhibit light brown, papery lesions on the leaf tips and edges. These lesions can eventually cover half the leaf but rarely the whole leaf. Mature plants will survive heat and drought injury with reduced yields; seedlings, however, may die. Irrigation has been used to arrest drought injury.

Chemical Injury

Application of high concentrations of fungicides or insecticides can cause plant disfigurement similar to fungus infections. Copper sulfate (without lime) can burn small brown holes in ginseng leaves. This speckling effect is very pronounced during hot weather. A Bordeaux mixture is safer, although it can also burn during extremely dry periods. Ridomil also burns ginseng plants at high application rates. These injuries appear as white searing along the leaf edges. Any chemical has the potential to damage ginseng plants, and all should be used at the lowest concentration possible to offer the necessary control.

DISEASE CONTROL

One of the most important concerns in ginseng cultivation is to keep disease out of the garden. All other problems pale in comparison to losing your entire crop. A lot of people think that natural-shade gardens are not very susceptible to disease, but that's just nor true. Don't allow anyone to smoke or use tobacco in or around your ginseng garden, as tobacco can carry diseases very similar to ginseng blights. I've also seen natural-shade gardens suffer horribly from Alternaria blight. In one case, about 90 percent of the wood-land ginseng plants were dying of Alternaria each July because the grower didn't spray. The disease never spread to the roots, so the next year the plants valiantly sprouted again, only to have the cycle repeat. With only two months' growth each year (May and June), the roots didn't get very big very fast.

Ginseng diseases are controlled by applying fungicides. Technically, fungicides must be labeled for ginseng to be used legally but few chemical controls are so labeled. A company wishing to label for a specific crop must conduct comprehensive studies into the potential for soil and groundwater contamination and residue in the product. That costs money. In the reality of agribusiness, companies cannot justify huge up-front expenses for small acreage crops like ginseng. It has been the practice of ginseng growers to use a wide variety of potato fungicides and insecticides while they wait for labeling to include ginseng. This is illegal, but it is a reality of the ginseng business. Growers using nonlabeled pesticides run the risk of having their roots confiscated if testing shows chemical residues in the product.

The Environmental Protection Agency (EPA) has a system in place called the IR-4 program to provide grant money for labeling small-acreage crops. It is currently being used in the Midwest to monitor ginseng disease and insect control applications. Several chemicals were approved in Wisconsin for use on ginseng in 1994. The list may change in future years, since chemical residue studies are currently under way for dried-root crops. Therefore, you should consult your state Agriculture Department to determine the status of approval and/or local restrictions for controls.

Fungicides and pesticides come in the form of wettable powder, dry flowable powder (DF), liquid concentrate, or dust. Wettable powders, dry flowable powders, and liquid concentrates are mixed with water and applied through a sprayer. Dry flowable powders are fairly recent improvements in the field, being slightly more granular than the older wettable powders and therefore easier to mix. Liquid concentrates are the easiest to mix, and the chemical tends to stay in suspension while in the sprayer tank. Powders settle out if the tank isn't shaken occasionally. Powders are usually less expensive than liquid concentrates.

Spreader-sticker solutions can be mixed with the chemicals to enhance coverage in two ways. They break the surface tension of the water molecules, causing the spray to "sheet" across the leaves, and they are also slightly tacky, which tends to hold the chemical barrier in place during a moderate misting. A small amount of dishwashing liquid, such as Ivory, can be added to the spray mixture as a low-cost spreader. Soaps act only as spreaders and not stickers, so they will not hold pesticides on the leaf if it rains.

Sprays are administered by mechanized equipment in commercial gardens and through backpack or garden sprayers on smaller plots. It is important to cover upper and lower leaf surfaces and stems completely in order to obtain the best protection. Most fungicides should also be applied to plants before disease becomes apparent. Dusts are applied with a duster, such as the Dustin Mizer.

Follow the proper mixing directions and do not overapply chemicals. Overapplication is costly and could harm both the plants and the environment. The dilution rates may be a little confusing at first to the small-plot cultivator, since they are often stated in pounds (or pints) per hundred gallons instead of tablespoons per gallon. When using smaller amounts, simply reduce the gallons from one hundred to ten or five and make the same percentage reduction in the chemical.

Use caution in handling any chemicals and follow instructions for using a respirator or other protective equipment. Also be aware that a person applying the spray may be a bit more sensitive to chemicals in the confines of a ginseng bed than in an open field where the testing was conducted.

Following are descriptions of the more common fungicides and pesticides that have been used on cultivated ginseng. Not all of the chemicals discussed are listed for ginseng, but all have been used over the years by growers. Remember to check with your state Agriculture Department to determine which controls are currently approved for use on ginseng.

Maneb is a generic name for a very good all-around stem and leaf blight fungicide commonly used on potatoes. It is a surface preventative spray, which means it prevents fungus spores from penetrating a plant's cells. As such, it must be in place on the leaf before spores are carried to the plant. It also has a benefit as a contact fungicide, killing inactive spores on the leaf's surface. It does not, however, kill fungus spores that have already penetrated the leaf. Commercial maneb mixes, such as Dithane and Manzate 200, also contain small amounts of zinc. Zinc can be toxic to ginseng in large amounts, but the small percentage in these fungicides is not. Maneb is used at ten- to fourteen-day intervals throughout the growing season and after heavy rainfalls or frequent leaf wettings.

Kocide and *Champion Wettable Powder* are brand names of *copper hydroxide,* another excellent fungicide. These fungicides, along with *Rovral,* tend to have the same general effect as maneb.

Captan is a surface preventative spray that has no effect other than to coat the plant surface and prevent spores from attacking. It does not kill fungus spores that have already alighted on the leaves. Captan is applied every ten to fourteen days through the growing season and after frequent wettings. It can be effective on ginseng, although many growers feel it is not as potent as maneb. Captan is commonly found in home orchard sprays. These orchard mixtures

PESTICIDES LABELED FOR USE
ON GINSENG IN WISCONSIN—1994

Pest	Materials
Alternaria	Champion Wettable Powder, Flowable Champ, Dithane DF, Aliette WDG, Rovral, Rovral 4 Flowable, Kocide 101, Kocide DF, Kocide LF
Phytophthora	Aliette WDG, Ridomil 5G, Ridomil 2E
Weed Control	Fusilade 2000, Fusilade DX
Soil Fumigants	Basamid, Vapam
Slugs	Deadline Bullets, Durham Metaldehyde Granules 7.5, Slug Pellets M-2
Insects	D.Z.N. Diazinon 14G, D.Z.N. Diazinon AG 500, Pyrenone Crop Spray

This list is provided only to show pesticides in use by commercial growers in Wisconsin in 1994. Most of these chemicals carried full federal labels and were legal for use anywhere in the United States at that time. Approved pesticides do change from year to year. Contact your state Agriculture Department or state university extension office for an updated list before using any pesticides on ginseng. Agriculture officials can get specific, up-to-date information on approved chemicals from the University of Wisconsin-Madison, Department of Plant Pathology.

are used by some small-plot growers because they contain an insecticide in addition to the fungicide.

Copper sulfate and *Bordeaux mixture* (named after the Bordeaux region in France, where it was developed for use on grapes) have also been reported as effective fungicides on ginseng. Copper sulfate has a tendency to burn small holes in ginseng leaves, so it is often mixed with hydrated lime to form a more mellow Bordeaux compound. Both copper sulfate and Bordeaux mixtures can be purchased at farm and garden stores.

Ridomil is a systemic fungicide, which means it is absorbed by and circulated throughout the plant. Developed for use on potatoes and tobacco, it is applied differently to each crop. Ridomil is upwardly mobile, meaning that it is most effectively translocated up through the root system. It does not move down very well, so any spray done on the leaves will move throughout the leaves and stem but not into the root. Therefore, for tobacco it is used in granular form on the soil surface in order to reach the roots, and for potatoes it is sprayed on the leaves so that the chemical does not contaminate the tuber.

As a foliar spray on ginseng, Ridomil is often used in combination with stem and leaf blight fungicides. For root rot, Ridomil is used as a soil drench (or as a top dressing in the granular form) so that the chemical agent leaches into the ground and reaches the roots.

Benlate and *Aliette* are additional systemic fungicides applied as a foliar spray. They are often used in conjunction with a stem and leaf blight fungicide.

With repeated use of certain fungicides, diseases may become resistant to the chemical control. For example, Ridomil-resistant Phytophthora root rot has been discovered in some areas. Natural shade, good sanitation, wide spacing, and dependable drainage can reduce the reliance on chemical controls and may help avoid resistance to control sprays.

INSECT CONTROL

Insects are generally not a significant problem on ginseng, but heavy damage can occur from local infestations of leafhoppers, tree crickets, aphids, and jumping plant lice. Jumping plant lice are notorious in some regions of the country for destroying up to 90 percent of a seed crop. Look for a cottony, mildewlike mass on the peduncle just under the flower head. Touch the cotton, and part of it will move. These pests suck the fluid from the flower stem, resulting in dull, mummified berries and lifeless seeds. Fortunately, several common insecticides are effective against jumping plant lice. Insecticides commonly used by growers are Sevin (carbaryl), Diazinon, Malathion, and Pyrenone, which is organic.

Insecticides are often mixed with fungicides so that a single application handles two chores. Insecticides, are not used every ten days like fungicides; only one to three applications of an insecticide are used per year unless specific problems require additional control. Foliar fertilizer can also be combined with fungicides and insecticides to add a feeding while managing insects and diseases. Contact your state Agriculture Department each year to determine which insecticides are approved for ginseng.

A private applicator's license may be required for chemical purchase and application. The program is administered by the EPA through state agriculture departments. Licenses and application requirements vary slightly from state to state. Contact your county extension agent for details on obtaining a private applicator's license if you need one to buy and apply chemical controls.

Root Knot Nematodes

Root knot nematodes are microscopic wormlike animals of the genus *Meloidogyne*. They can be found on ginseng in many regions but are more prevalent in warmer climates and do the most damage in sandy soils. Plants infected with root knot nematodes may appear stunted, wilt, or show discolored foliage. The roots display galls, often on the smaller fiber roots, which house the adult nematodes. The larvae live in the soil. Nematodes can result in misshapen roots and reduced yields, but mature roots are often marketable if the galls are trimmed away.

Avoid soils known to contain nematodes and don't bring in soil from another location for use in your ginseng beds. Since no nematicides are labeled for ginseng and no widespread studies have been undertaken, it is unknown if nematicides are effective for control in ginseng gardens.

Slugs and Snails

Slugs and snails are common land mollusks that find ginseng seeds quite appetizing. They will crawl under the mulch and happily eat the core out of every seed they find. Slugs also feast on the necks or buds of ginseng roots that stick above ground level. They do not dig, so anything buried is relatively safe. They are enough of a threat, however, that most commercial growers place slug bait poison out before seeding.

RODENTS AND OTHER PESTS

Mice, voles, and chipmunks are also very fond of ginseng seeds and roots. They not only eat maturing seeds on the plant but will follow a row of freshly sown seeds and dig out every nugget they can find. Chipmunks are considered by many growers to be the worst pest on the seed crop. Mice and voles attack maturing roots by following mole tunnels through the ginseng garden and gnawing on the roots that are exposed. Moles themselves can cause considerable damage, not because they eat ginseng roots, but because they tunnel right through the roots looking for subterranean insects and worms. Larger ginseng roots will recover from mole damage, but their value is drastically reduced.

Rodenticides can be placed around the garden in covered bait stations (a plastic pipe lying on its side will suffice) to reduce rodent damage. Trapping may be more ecologically sound, however, since owls that eat poisoned rodents can also become sick. Moles can be caught with traps or poisoned. A few woodland growers position aluminum sheeting as a barrier around the entire perimeter of their gardens. The aluminum is buried several inches deep to deter burrowing animals while leaving a foot or more protruding above ground to stop small animals from entering the garden. Rodents inside the plot are either trapped or poisoned, and the aluminum wall prevents reinfestation.

Just about any critter that can get into the ginseng garden is likely to be considered a pest. These include groundhogs, rabbits, deer, and cattle. Some of these animals will eat the ginseng plants, and all will trample them. In either circumstance, growth is stopped for the rest of the year on damaged plants. Rabbits have a particularly nasty habit of hopping through ginseng beds and nipping off stalks, leaving behind a trail of uneaten herbage. Growers who blaze away at rabbits in the garden, however, sometimes find that the shotgun pellets destroy more ginseng leaves than the bunnies do!

A few growers let a cat or ferret handle small pest control in enclosed gardens. I know one grower who claims the mere scent of a ferret keeps rodents at bay, so his pest control consists of taking his pet ferret for a weekly romp around the ginseng garden. Foxes and owls are excellent mousers and may offer natural control in many woodland settings. Foxes can present a bit of a problem around newly sown plots since they love to dig in freshly turned earth. Still, a few bare spots in the ginseng garden are a small price to pay for year-around rodent control and the chance to glimpse a sleek red fox on the prowl for his dinner.

In regions where deer or elk are a nuisance, fencing is a common method of keeping them out of the ginseng plot. A less costly trick for repelling members of the deer family is to place bars of deodorant soap in hosiery and hang them around the garden.

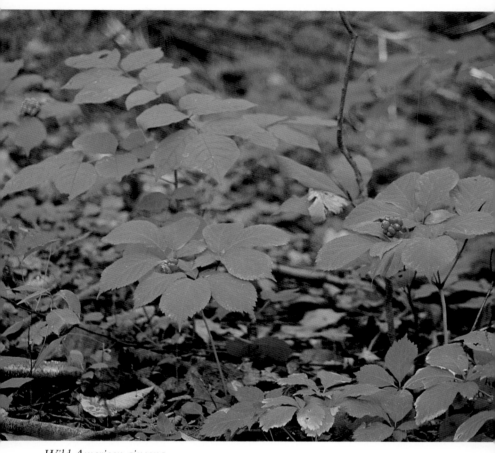

*Wild American ginseng
in its natural habitat.*

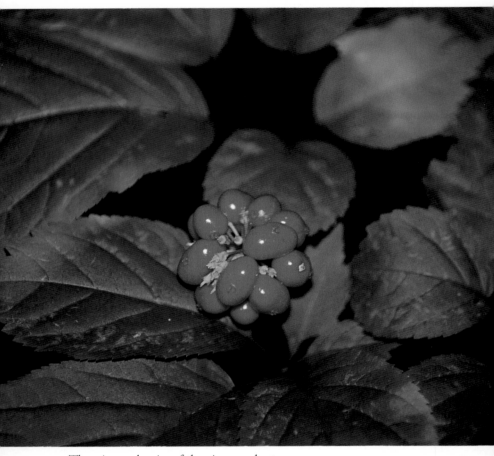

*The crimson berries of the ginseng plant
hold from one to three seeds. Diggers have
a legal and moral responsibility to plant all
wild seeds back into the wild.*

One-year-old ginseng plants under wood-lathe shade. Note how excess moisture drains away from the raised beds into trenches.

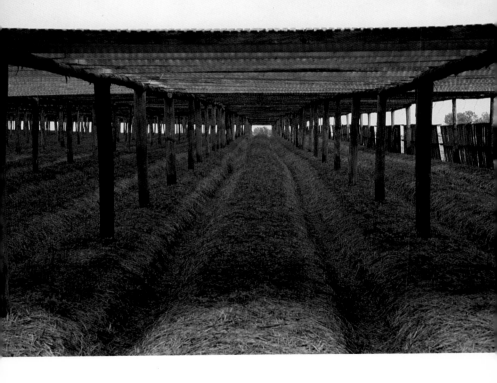

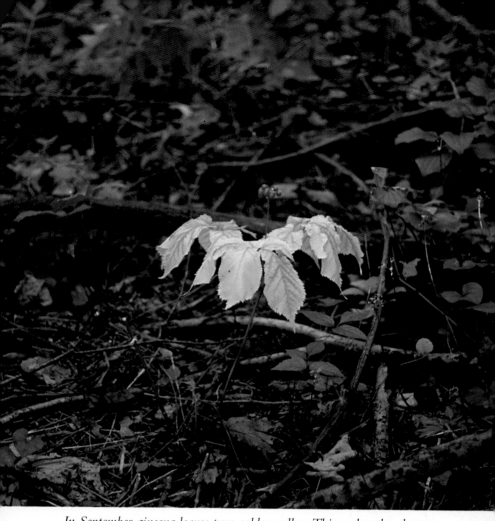

In September, ginseng leaves turn golden yellow. This makes the plant easy to spot in the forest undergrowth.

A one-year-old root (top) compared to a seven-year-old woodsgrown root (bottom). The older root is stout and well ringed—desirable qualities in a ginseng root. (photo by J. L. Pritts)

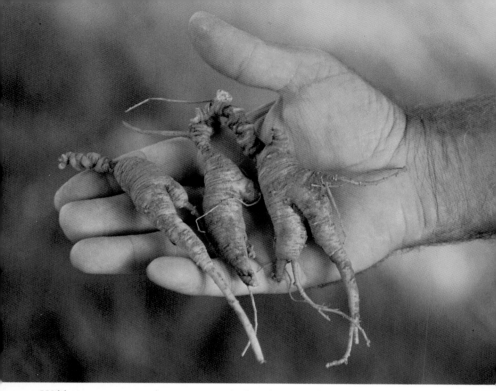

Wild ginseng roots as large as a man's thumb are good, harvestable roots.

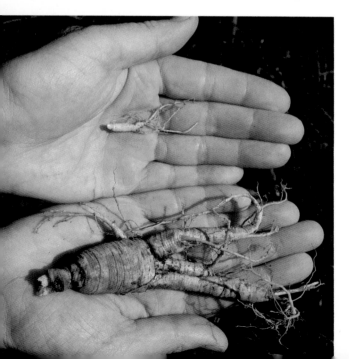

From left to right: a four-year-old artificial-shade root, a nine-year-old wild-simulated root, a twenty-year-old wild root.

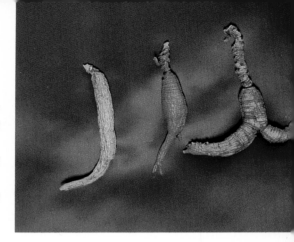

Counting the cup-shaped bud scars on a ginseng root's neck will reveal the age of the plant—one scar for each year of growth.

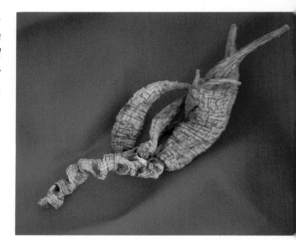

"Deer horn" roots (left) and "octopus" roots (right) are of little value.

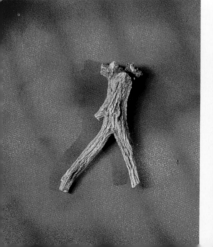

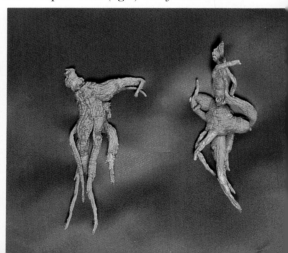

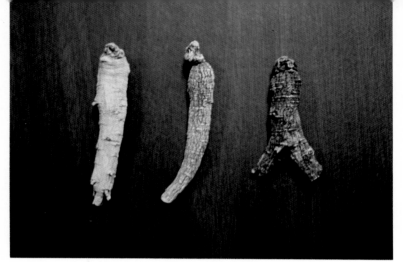

Cultivated roots show the varying colors of dried ginseng. The root on the left is too clean and white; the middle root is of good color for field-cultivated ginseng; the root on the right is the color that is currently in demand for woodsgrown and wild-simulated ginseng.

These cultivated roots that have been trimmed by professionals have creamy white interiors; several show a dark center, however, indicating improper drying. Diggers and cultivators should never trim roots.

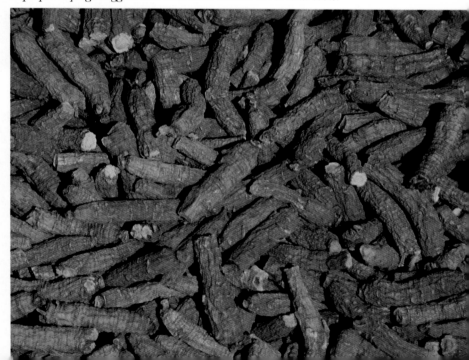

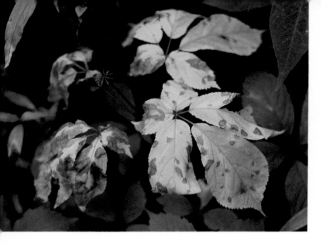

This woodland ginseng plant is suffering from severe Alternaria blight.

This sunburned ginseng plant will die if additional shade is not erected.

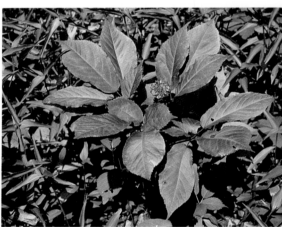

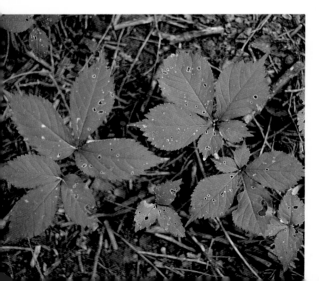

One- and two-year-old ginseng plants. The circular holes in the leaves were caused by insects or tiny slugs. The seedling in the lower center has a small Alternaria lesion on one leaf; note the tell-tale yellow halo surrounding the lesion.

Chapter 6

Harvesting and Marketing

These Tartars every year, either as subjects or friends, came into China by the Province of Leotung to traffic with the inhabitants . . . the merchandise they brought were several, as the root called ginsem, so much esteemed amongst the Chineses, and all sorts of precious skins.

Martinus Martini,
London, 1654

Afther the ginseng has been cultivated and grown, or if you have found a good source of the root in the wild, the next concern is proper harvesting and marketing.

SEED HARVEST

The first harvest from your ginseng garden will be the fruit—berries containing seeds. Three-year-old and older plants produce crimson berries each year in late summer and early fall. Each berry holds from one to three seeds, with two being most common. Some two-year-old plants yield a few berries, but they are not reliable producers.

Seed production slows the growth of the ginseng root, since the plant uses much of its nutrition in producing offspring. Root weight can increase dramatically over a period of a few years in plants that are not permitted to produce berries. Some growers snip the flower buds of many of their plants during the spring to stop berry formation and force the growth into the roots. Although a bit time consuming, this is an excellent idea for the grower who needs only enough seeds to sustain the next year's planting.

Seeds are a valuable harvest for commercial growers, since they currently command a higher price per pound than cultivated ginseng roots. And unlike roots, which can be harvested only once from a single plant, seeds are produced each year from the third year on. For the small grower, however, seed sales are unlikely to generate much income after paying for advertising, handling, shipping, and the occasional bad check. Also, putting more seed on the market might reduce the future value of ginseng roots as more growers enter the business and send their roots to market.

Berries ripen over a period of several weeks, with the fruit at lower and outer portions of the plant ripening first. It is wise to pick berries as they ripen under natural shade since chipmunks, mice, and birds will also be eyeing the inviting red treats.

The seeds inside the freshly picked berries are called green, or unstratified, seeds. Since ginseng seeds have an eighteen-month dormant period during which they must remain moist, most growers stratify the seeds by burying them in damp sand for a year. Some woodland growers forgo stratification and simply plant the green seed soon after it is picked: This closely simulates the natural dispersal of wild ginseng seeds. It cuts down on labor and seed handling but puts the seeds at risk of predation from forest animals and birds. It also ties up a garden plot for an extra year.

Seeds can be depulped before stratification, or whole berries can be placed in sand—the pulp will disintegrate within a month or two, leaving behind the seeds. Some growers believe this invites bacteria to form on the seeds, while others report good success with this method. Many large-scale growers run their berries through depulping machines or mash the berries in cloth sacks and hang them until the pulp has fermented and disintegrated. Holding the berries for a few days after harvest softens the fruit and makes for easier seed removal with either method.

After pulp removal, seeds are water-tested. To do this, simply pour the seeds into a large bucket of water and skim off the ones that float—these are not viable and must be discarded. The good seeds should be air dried for a brief period in a shaded spot and then mixed with damp, but not wet, sand for stratification. Growers are divided on whether it is better to layer green seeds in the sand or simply mix them in. Either method is acceptable, using about three parts sand to one part seed. The seed/sand mixture is placed in a screen-mesh box, buried in a shaded location, and covered with dirt. The box must have a screened top and bottom so that water can drain through naturally. Seed boxes should not be buried too deeply in order to maintain good drainage. Many growers set their boxes in very shallow impressions and mound dirt over them. The seeds will remain underground, experiencing the natural warm-cold cycles of nature until the following autumn, when they will be unearthed and planted in garden beds. Any seeds that jump the gun and sprout in only six months will be lost in the stratification box.

When the boxes of sand and seed are unearthed, the seeds can easily be recovered by spraying a stream of water through the screen. This washes away the sand and leaves clean seeds ready for planting.

Since eighteen months is a long time to wait for ginseng seeds to sprout, some studies have been done on compressing two years' worth of nature's cold/warm cycles into one. Forced growth has largely been unsuccessful in these attempts. Growers have also experimented with keeping seeds in an extended summer condition for six months (July through December) instead of a hot and cold sequence in the same period. The theory is that the imperfect embryo inside the kernel might develop enough during this time to sprout the following spring. Interestingly, the Koreans pick their seeds in July and August, pack them in sand, and keep them at about sixty-eight degrees through November. At that time, the seeds that have split are planted and those that have not are discarded. This practice of using only dehiscent seeds tends to produce generations of early-germinating parent stock, and the Koreans have an excellent first-year success rate with their seeds. Southern growers have also found that up to 40 percent of their seeds sprout the first spring when handled in such a manner.

Others trying to give Mother Nature a nudge have used chemical plant hormones. Some success has been reported in stimulating ginseng seeds to germinate within six months through the use of potassium gibberellate, but many batches of seeds have been lost this way, because a bit too much of the chemical causes the seed to burst and too little yields an inconsequential germination rate.

It's best to stick with the natural eighteen-month method of seed handling. Realistically, the storage period is relatively unimportant in the cycle after two seed crops have been harvested and stored.

If desired, seeds can be treated with a fungicide before placement in a stratification box or upon removal from the box. Fungicides can prevent the spread of disease on the seeds but may also reduce seed viability somewhat. Reduced viability usually only occurs when too much chemical agent is used in the solution. Fungicide treatment for seeds is covered in chapter 4.

ROOTS

Roots are generally harvested after four growing seasons under artificial shade, after six to eight years for woodsgrown roots, and after eight to fifteen years for wild-simulated ginseng. Roots are dug as the plants begin to die down in the fall. The roots are heaviest at this time, since the strength from the withering plant has been concentrated in the root.

How many roots will you harvest from your plot? Commercial growers aim for one ton of dried roots (about three and a half tons fresh) per acre under artificial shade after four or five years. Under natural shade, the rule of thumb is a maximum of about half a ton of dried roots (about one and three-quarter ton fresh) after six years. Woodsgrown crops produce a lower yield because of wider plant spacing and competition for nutrients from trees. Fall-dug ginseng roots lose about 65 to 70 percent of their weight after drying. Spring-dug roots lose even more, up to 80 percent. As a general rule, it takes about three and a half pounds of fall-harvested or five pounds of spring-harvested roots to make one pound dried. Roots are harvested in the spring only if a severe disease outbreak threatens to destroy the entire crop before autumn.

Several methods are used to harvest ginseng, from using

mechanical diggers to hand digging each root. Just about anybody who has ever turned shovelfuls of dirt in the ginseng garden eventually tinkers with the idea of creating the perfect mechanized ginseng digger. Large-scale growers use modified potato diggers under artificial shade but find these difficult to operate in woodland gardens because of the tree roots that invade the garden over the years. Smaller natural-shade growers generally stick with the laborious task of digging by hand. It may take as many as 200 hours to harvest a quarter-acre plot under natural shade.

Ginseng roots should be handled carefully, since much of their value is in their shape. The roots must be removed intact insofar as it is humanly possible. Cuts or breaks in the roots will reduce their value.

A digging fork or a shovel can be used in hand digging, although a fork tends to cut roots less. With either implement, start at one end of a bed by digging in below the root level and prying up. It is best to continue in a line, setting the shovel in from the toe of the overturned dirt and prying up a new batch of dirt and roots. It is helpful to rake the mulch from the beds before digging.

Very small roots should be set aside and replanted within a few days. Small roots will lower the value of your entire batch, so they are much more valuable as transplanted seed producers than as dried tubers. They can be harvested for market after two or more additional years of growth.

Roots must be rinsed, but not right away. Through proper root cleaning, a digger or cultivator can make good roots even better. Rule number one: Asians like dirt in the rings of the roots. Personally, I'm quite happy to sell them all the dirt they want at $300 a pound. The roots should be rinsed but not cleaned.

Always let your roots dry for a few days with dirt attached before rinsing. This will allow the roots to darken. Asians tend to like a fairly dark root in woodsgrown ginseng and a more straw-colored root in field-cultivated ginseng. Wild root color should be somewhere in between. This is for freshly rinsed roots; the roots naturally turn a little darker and duller as they dry.

If your roots come out of the garden clean and nearly white, you might have to add some dirt. Mix up a bucket of mud and dump it over your white roots. Stir the roots around so they are coated with muck, then pull them out and let them dry for several days.

After several days of wilting, the roots will be ready to rinse. Everyone develops his or her own technique for rinsing roots; I toss them into a big tub of clean water and swish them around until they look right. That's about all there is to it. I do check the roots as I put them on a drying rack. If any are a bit too dirty, I run water over them and rub off the excess dirt with my thumb. Other growers use a variety of methods for rinsing their roots, from low-pressure sprayers to a few turns in a washing machine. Whatever the procedure, roots must not be overcleaned. White roots bring a very low price.

Drying ginseng roots to perfection is considered an art by many. The basic principle is to get the roots to ninety to one hundred degrees Fahrenheit and remove the humidity from the surrounding air. A good slow dry at ninety degrees for ten to fourteen days will bring roots to the point at which they break with a crisp snap under pressure and show a creamy-white interior. Drying too quickly can scorch roots and create a pronounced green or brown discoloration inside the root when broken. Drying too slowly or failing to control the humidity can invite mildew and dark mold spots on the root's exterior.

When the process is done correctly, the roots become very limp after the first few days, then gradually shrink, shrivel, and stiffen. Since ginseng roots lose 65 to 70 percent of their weight in drying, the change in size will be dramatic. Smaller roots dry quickly, while larger roots take a few extra days to harden.

Commercial growers stack racks of screens in drying huts or trailers and spread a single layer of roots on each screen. The huts have some type of heat source and are equipped with a vent and fan high in the wall to expel humidity. Some growers start each fresh batch of roots on the lower screens, then move them up one rack each day until they reach the top, at which time they are dry. This allows for a continuous supply of roots to be dug and dried, spreading the harvest out over many days. It's also an easy way to keep track of the drying time of each batch.

Small-plot cultivators might also use drying huts but often transform top-floor or attic rooms into drying chambers during September of each year. Closed off with a fan and dehumidifier running, these drying rooms are fairly effective if the temperature remains high. Ginseng roots will dry just about anyplace where a toasty warm temperature and low humidity can be maintained. Microwave ovens, however, are not acceptable for drying ginseng.

Since I don't grow ginseng on a large scale, I'm able to use the natural heat in my modest attic for drying. I don't have a drying shed, although I sometimes close the windows on my garden shed and let the heat build up in order to dry my ginseng. One thing to avoid is drying ginseng in direct sunlight. It doesn't draw out the root's moisture in the slow, even fashion that is required. Another thing to avoid is stacking piles of ginseng on a screen, since dry air must be able to circulate freely and gently draw moisture out of the roots. Roots that touch might develop moldy spots. Place only a single layer of roots on a screen. Stacking screens several inches apart is okay.

Extended periods of damp weather in late September can cause problems because ginseng roots definitely develop mildew and rot spots when the temperature falls and the humidity rises. If the weather turns bad during drying, I simply move my ginseng down into various warm spots around the house. On one occasion I turned an unused bedroom into a drying room. With the heat turned up and a dehumidifier running, it worked just fine.

Dried roots are most often stored in fiberboard containers. The roots will absorb moisture from the air during clammy weather and must be able to breathe in order to keep from spoiling. Cardboard boxes or drums are ideal containers and should be kept in dry areas for long term storage. Once ginseng roots are dried, they can be held indefinitely at room temperature or cooler. Some growers have been known to hold their roots for several years, waiting for the price to go up.

MARKETING

A small percentage of American ginseng is sold to American manufacturers for use in capsules, teas, and cosmetics, but most of it is traded overseas. Some cultivated American ginseng goes to Chinatowns in the United States, but Chinese Americans don't buy a lot of wild root. They just don't have the time and expertise to grade it. The exported roots go to several different areas, including Hong Kong, Taiwan, Malaysia, and Singapore.

The first level in marketing ginseng overseas is the importer into the foreign country. Some American companies have overseas offices, so they act as exporters from the United States and importers into the receiving country. After arrival in Hong Kong, for example, the roots are auctioned to a grader. The graders come to the auction, purchase ginseng roots, and then grade them and sell them to stores.

In North America, the price of ginseng fluctuates somewhat over the course of a year, and selling a large lot at the right time can make for a hefty profit. Although there is no clear-cut rule on selling forest gold, most growers peddle their crop from October through December. Ginseng fever runs high in Wisconsin's Marathon County during this time of the year. Late-autumn visitors to

WILD GINSENG STATE CERTIFIED (pounds)

State	1988	1989	1990	1991	1992	1993
Alabama	795	1,034	585	779	1,774	1,037
Arkansas	4,124	4,054	2,666	2,730	5,295	2,582
Georgia	497	450	447	717	1,137	353
Illinois	3,607	6932	14,048	6,043	8,680	—
Indiana	6,748	11,698	11,670	5,283	13,645	10,459
Iowa	709	1,618	2,159	1,802	2,379	1,874
Kentucky	24,295	14,425	25,286	25,697	26,485	26,508
Maryland	65	128	198	105	105	175
Minnesota	1,650	2,190	2,138	1,770	2,390	—
Missouri	2,669	2,814	2,357	2,865	4,404	2,505
New York	1,175	259	478	493	—	—
North Carolina	7,743	4,111	6,415	9,056	9,691	9,674
Ohio	8,151	8,279	10,811	7,236	12,155	7,694
Pennsylvania	1,291	1,756	2,454	2,534	4,053	—
Tennessee	21,129	18,701	12,522	16,338	25,299	13,840
Vermont	295	247	378	407	398	0
Virginia	8,664	8,375	10,167	13,134	13,148	10,075
West Virginia	15,384	14,407	15,991	18,808	23,226	19,224
Wisconsin	2,826	3,915	4,447	4,007	5,235	4,075
Totals	111,817	105,393	125,217	119,804	159,499	110,075

Includes only ginseng certified for export and not necessarily the entire production of the state. Courtesy of U.S. Fish & Wildlife Service.

the region may be surprised by vanloads of Hong Kong buyers barreling down country roads, shouting Chinese into cellular phones, and leaving swirling leaves and snowflakes in their wake. U.S. buyers are busy also, sealing $100,000 deals with a handshake and a smile before darting off to other barnyards full of dried and drying roots of gold.

CULTIVATED GINSENG STATE CERTIFIED (pounds)

State	1988	1989	1990	1991	1992	1993
Alabama	45	0	0	1	16	0
Arkansas	114	0	56	0	0	0
Georgia	795	1,059	797	249	711	286
Illinois	2,525	3,460	6,526	387	2,090	—
Indiana	866	600	362	344	317	440
Iowa	114	21	10	11	803	19
Kentucky	2,185	958	2,471	2,685	1,815	116
Maryland	824	291	2,150	762	762	1,509
Minnesota	1,582	1,901	3,206	6,118	3,833	—
Missouri	27	290	220	17	28	9
New York	721	0	0	727	—	—
North Carolina	797	175	792	317	496	24
Ohio	43	177	0	89	69	113
Pennsylvania	192	689	238	2,196	24	—
Tennessee	5,116	6,670	6,313	6,616	1,278	5,304
Vermont	308	4,380	4,770	3,952	0	308
Virginia	459	763	715	674	1,371	175
West Virginia	109	25	200	659	1,229	611
Wisconsin	1,041,241	1,356,505	1,341,535	1,160,874	1,634,227	1,371,392
Totals	1,058,063	1,377,964	1,370,361	1,186,678	1,649,069	1,380,306

Includes only ginseng certified for export and not necessarily the entire production of the state. Courtesy of U.S. Fish & Wildlife Service.

Those who live outside the ginseng capital of the United States are unlikely to be called upon in person by a ginseng dealer and therefore must find a buyer for their roots. Many ginseng dealers advertise in outdoor magazines such as *Fur-Fish-Game* and *The Trapper and Predator Caller.*

Dealing with a ginseng buyer can be handled in several ways.

On small lots—less than three pounds of wild and twenty pounds of cultivated—the roots are usually shipped on faith to a buyer and the price paid for the roots is accepted by the seller. Since a reputable buyer will give you the best price available at the time, you don't need to be concerned about being taken on small lots. Another way to handle small lots—generally limited to wild roots—is to sell to a roving country buyer. This is usually a cash deal but often results in a lower price for the goods than might have been realized by selling to a major dealer.

A third method is to send several pounds of a large lot as a sample and ask for a price quote. This is a good method for woods-grown and wild-simulated ginseng, since a buyer adept at grading will offer a higher price for the better-quality roots. Most buyers can differentiate between wild and artificial-shade-cultivated roots; the real problem occurs in determining the value of woodsgrown and wild-simulated. An uncertain buyer will always downgrade the roots in order to make certain he covers his costs. A buyer who recognizes the true value of woodsgrown and wild-simulated can offer a higher price—much higher in some cases. If the quote is acceptable, the entire lot is shipped. As long as the sample is representative of the entire shipment, the agreed-upon price will be paid. Understandably, problems will arise if a grower offers only his best roots for a price quote and then ships a large parcel of inferior roots for the sale. A lower price should always be expected in this circumstance, and a grower who earns a reputation for mixing roots should expect low bids for future crops.

Different grades of ginseng should not be mixed. This doesn't mean you have to know the scores of grades of ginseng recognized in the Orient, only that you keep wild and cultivated roots separate during a sale. If different types of roots are shipped in one container, they must be secured in separate, clearly labeled packages inside the shipping container. Also, don't ship debris such as twigs and stems in the parcels. This rubble must be removed by the buyer before weighing and might influence him or her to grade your roots somewhat harshly. Don't resort to trickery to add weight or upgrade your roots. Buyers know all about drilled out roots filled with BBs or roots that have had threads tied around them during drying in an effort to add more rings. Plan on receiving a very low price for your entire lot if this type of chicanery is discovered.

Roots should be shipped in a sturdy cardboard container with plenty of cushioning material, such as wadded newspaper or foam peanuts. Double-boxing is a good idea, as is placing the roots inside a paper bag within the box. If the box is broken open in transit, the roots will be contained within the bag. The longer necks of the older roots will be particularly susceptible to breakage during shipping, so careful packaging is a must.

The U.S. Postal Service and other delivery services such as UPS will deliver boxes of ginseng roots. Check weight and size restrictions for packages before shipping. UPS currently will deliver packages up to 150 pounds through their regular interstate service. That's good news if you have 150 pounds of ginseng but bad news if you're sending a small box of fragile roots. A large carton might end up atop your precious cargo in a bouncing, swaying truck. Cushion your package accordingly.

Although cultivated ginseng can be marketed at any time, many states have regulations on when wild ginseng can be bought and sold. This regulation may apply to woodsgrown and wild-cultivated roots as well. Some states, such as Pennsylvania, require anyone shipping ginseng roots out of the state to obtain a buyer's license for certification purposes, even if the person is only a cultivator or wild-ginseng digger and not a buyer. Cultivators and 'sangers are limited to selling within the state unless they fork over $50 for a buyer's license each year. The Natural Resources or Agriculture Department of your state should be able to provide you with current regulation information regarding harvest, selling, and time limitations.

Chapter 7

Hunting and Conserving Wild Ginseng

Ginseng is not everywhere very common, for sometimes you may search the woods for a space of several miles without finding a single plant of it . . . many people fear lest by continuing for several successive years to collect these plants without leaving one or two in each place to propagate their species, there will soon be very few of them left; which I think is likely to happen, for by all accounts they formerly grew in abundance round Montreal, but at present there is not a single plant of it to be found, so effectually have they been rooted out.

Peter Kalm, Swedish naturalist
studying Canadian flora,
7 August 1749

Within a decade after Kalm penned those words, wild American ginseng was nearly extinct in Canada. That's why smart 'sangers are conservationists, not opportunists. They know that conserving wild ginseng makes economic—as well as ecological—sense. Not everyone has gotten this message, however. Some uninformed diggers ferret out every ginseng plant they can find, regardless of size or season. Ginseng cannot survive under that kind of harvest pressure. Therefore, federal and state agencies have developed ginseng harvest regulations for most of the states within the natural range of wild ginseng. These regulations are intended to keep our native ginseng from following the path of its Asian cousin, wild *Panax ginseng.*

Wild Asian ginseng had become so rare by the early 1900s that a ginseng digger might search for days to find a single mature plant. Russian explorer and traveler Nikolai Apollonovich Baikov (1872–1958) discovered the dedication required to harvest wild ginseng in Asia when he accompanied a venerable Chinese ginseng hunter in 1910. Crossing and recrossing a steep wooded valley along the Lian-tsu River, the old Chinese 'sanger zeroed in on a particular ravine and there the two men spent several days methodically searching for the elusive plant. Finally Baikov recorded the discovery of a single ginseng plant, "among the heavy thickets of bracken and wood sorrel." During several additional weeks of hunting, the Russian adventurer and Chinese digger were able to find only three harvestable roots of wild Asian ginseng. Following are some of Nickolai Baikov's observations about the Asian ginseng hunters of an earlier era, and of their devotion to the hunt for wild ginseng:

> The plant's rarity and high price for which it is sold in China have produced a special type of ginseng hunter. In general they are people with neither hearth nor home who, to earn their livelihood, have had to live in the remote

forest. Their dress and equipment are an oiled apron which protects them from the dew, a long stick with which to part the leaves and grasses, a wooden bracelet on the left arm, and a badger skin hanging behind from their belt which lets them sit on wet ground. They generally wear a conical hat of birch bark, tied under the chin by a thong, and shoes of tarred pigskin.

Every year the ginseng hunters go off into the depths of the taiga. They go each their separate ways, rarely in pairs, not carrying arms, strong only in their prayers and the firm belief that the forest and mountain spirits will come to their aid in their undertaking. They spend the night wherever evening finds them, taking shelter in a cave or under a rock if it rains, but passing most nights under the stars, sleeping near a fire on the old badger skin. Sometimes these poor men die of hunger, often they fall victim to the great beasts of the taiga, tigers, panthers, and bears.

These obstacles and dangers do not lessen the courage and perseverance of the ginseng hunter. They believe all these dangers exist only to frighten away cowards, to turn them away from the places where the ginseng grows. In the minds of the Chinese, only a pure and virtuous man can find the root of life. The immoral man would never know how to succeed there, for the plant disappears at his approach and the root sinks deep into the earth; from the undergrowth springs the ginseng's guardian, the tiger, and he devours the misguided adventurer.

When the hunter finds a plant, he throws aside his stick, covers his eyes and says a prayer to the divinity. He studies the place of discovery with great care; the lay of the land, the kind of soil, neighboring plants, the plant's situation with regard to sun and wind—everything is taken into consideration. Then the hunter examines the plant itself and digs away the earth to expose the root for study. By this he determines its value, and if he finds it is still too small, he lets it live two or three more years, putting everything back in place and watering the plant to repay it for the trouble he has caused.

If the plant is thought worth digging, that operation is done with the help of special small spades made of bone. The gathered roots are usually put in a basket of birch bark, after being carefully wrapped in thin paper. The upper part of the plant, stem and leaves are not simply thrown away, but for superstitious reasons are burned. Any seeds are replanted.

Today's hunt for American ginseng is not quite so arduous as it was for the Chinese of yore, but it is still undertaken in much the same manner as in our own pioneer days. Modern technology has little effect on this part of our heritage. The ginseng hunter simply walks through forests searching for ginseng plants.

LEGAL REQUIREMENTS

Your first responsibility as a contemporary ginseng forager is to become aware of the legal restrictions in the states where you will be hunting ginseng. Contact the appropriate state environmental agency for information on digging permits, seasons, special permits for state-controlled lands, and digging on private property. Keep in mind that it may be a criminal violation in your state to dig ginseng on private land without permission of the landowner.

Ginseng is afforded federal protection by the Convention on International Trade in Endangered Species of Wild Fauna and Flora, 27 U.S.T. 108. A federal export permit is required for international trade. A permit can be secured only if the export will not have a detrimental effect on the species. The U.S. Fish and Wildlife Service is responsible for issuing permits and monitoring ginseng populations in the United States. In order to do this, the USFWS requires states in the natural range of ginseng to establish an acceptable ginseng protection program.

To qualify for federal recognition of their ginseng programs, states must have regulations in place to ensure that the ginseng populations under their control will not be harmed by harvest. The most common regulations establish a digging season after the berries have ripened, require the planting of all wild seeds near the parent plant, and limit the harvest to mature roots. Since ginseng harvest is a solitary endeavor, these restrictions are only effective in ensuring the survival of ginseng if diggers police their own ranks and follow the legal restrictions conscientiously.

Pennsylvania's ginseng regulations reflect the restrictions required by the federal mandate. Violations of these state regulations carry a fine of up to $100 for each ginseng plant illegally taken. Following is an excerpt of Pennsylvania's ginseng regulations as published in 25 Pennsylvania Code:

1. A person may harvest ginseng plants from August 1 through November 30.

2. Only mature ginseng plants with at least three leaves of five leaflets each may be harvested and only when the seeds (berries) are red.

3. Persons harvesting ginseng plants shall plant the seeds from the plant in the immediate vicinity of the collection site.

4. A person may not possess harvested, green ginseng roots between April 1 and August 1 of a calendar year.

Keep in mind that each state's regulations vary slightly. The digger must obtain and follow the regulations for each state in which he or she will be digging wild ginseng.

EQUIPMENT

You'll need very little equipment to enjoy the sport of 'sangin'. One handy tool is a walking stick. It can help you up steep slopes or become a snake prod for checking under rock ledges and fallen trees. Some 'sangers combine a digging implement with their walking stick by fastening a small spade to the bottom of the stick. A functional digging tool can be made by fastening a piece of metal pipe to the walking stick, then cutting one side of the extended pipe lengthwise and laying it open like a miniature shovel. A large screwdriver is the preferred digging tool for many 'sangers, since more prying than actual digging is involved in extricating wild roots. A common garden trowel is quite suitable as well.

A sack for carrying harvested roots rounds out the 'sanger's equipment—a plastic bread bag tucked under the belt and left hanging from the digger's side works well. A standard bread bag full of fresh ginseng roots will give you about a pound in dry weight, so it's a handy measuring device. It also holds moisture in the roots in case you are transplanting a few roots to a different location. I find that an unprotected plastic bag takes a lot of abuse from brambles, so I often carry a fanny pack or backpack and place the plastic bag inside of that. The pack is also handy for carrying a light lunch and a first-aid kit.

Wear comfortable clothing suitable to the climactic conditions in your region. Light-colored clothing is helpful in tick-infested tracts, since the little critters are a lot easier to see crawling across a khaki shirt than on a dark camouflaged jacket. Good hiking boots are a must in order to avoid a sprained ankle. If archery or rifle hunting seasons are open during the ginseng season, wearing a blaze orange hat is a prudent precaution.

SELECTING A HUNTING AREA
Once common throughout the eastern and midwestern United States, particularly in the Appalachian Mountains, wild ginseng has been picked over throughout its range. Patches of wild ginseng are

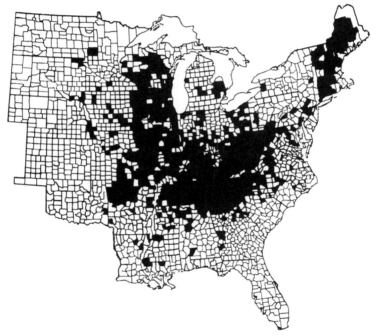

This map, compiled by the International Convention Advisory Commission in 1981, shows many of the counties where wild ginseng is reported to grow. Although the commission was disbanded before the map could be completed, the information does reveal the wide distribution of ginseng in the United States.

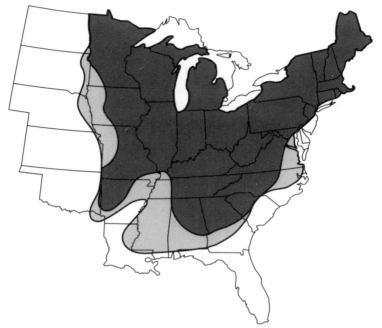

The darker shaded area represents an 1898 assessment of the wild ginseng range in the United States. In 1981, the International Convention Advisory Commission expanded the range to the lighter shaded area.

usually widely scattered, and locating a foraging area can be frustrating for the novice digger. Don't count on other 'sangers for help; they probably won't reveal their favorite ginseng hunting grounds. I've only found one secret foragers protect more: the location of their choice morel mushroom beds!

Ginseng is found in hardwood forests, so much of the eastern and midwestern hardwood forest area is potential ginseng habitat. In addition to the need for deciduous shade, soil type is important. If you find plenty of oak trees and mountain laurel, it is unlikely that you'll find ginseng. A slightly milder soil is to ginseng's liking, so start your search in areas of mixed maple, hickory, beech, and poplar with some oak. Swampy areas are out, as are dry ridge tops. Look for ginseng in rich forest loam, and don't discount rocky areas. Soil containing rocks the size of baseballs or larger discourages moles from tunneling, and nice patches of ginseng can sometimes be found in this coarse soil. The nicest wild ginseng grows in a moist to moderately dry soil, often where the sunlight seems almost too bright. When I find a forest clearing with a blackberry patch, I'm like a kid in a candy store. I dive in, crawling and picking my way through, and usually exit with a few scratches and some wild ginseng roots that would make your eyes bug out.

The ability to recognize ginseng's companion plants is a real bonus. Once you become adept at spotting good weeds like black cohosh, blue cohosh, Indian turnip, trillium, and wild sarsaparilla, you'll eventually run onto some ginseng. Some of these plants tolerate sunlight better than ginseng, and wild sarsaparilla tends to grow in drier soil than ginseng, but wild ginseng can often be found near these plants when the shade is favorable.

I sometimes slam on the brakes while driving and quickly pull to the berm in order to check out good weeds. I've found several patches of ginseng in this manner, some no more than a few steps from the well-traveled portion of a highway. An old-time digger also gave me this tip—ginseng grows best under the "soft" hardwoods, which are the first trees to turn color each autumn. He claims he can find good ginseng habitat by driving around in September and looking for splotches of red and yellow on otherwise green hillsides.

FORAGING

Choosing the proper time of the year for foraging is important. Ginseng roots are heaviest just as the plants die down in the fall, yet the plants must be standing for you to locate them. September is the best time of the year to dig wild ginseng. The roots are heavy, the berries are ripe, and the ginseng leaves start to turn a yellow-gold color that makes them fairly easy to spot.

Ginseng may grow alone or in family groups called patches. A typical ginseng patch will include all year classes of plants, from four-prongers down to the tiny tri-leaf seedlings. You will be interested in harvesting only the larger plants with three or more prongs. Small three-prongers will usually have small roots and should not be harvested. You can get some indication of root size by looking at the plant stalk. Slender stalks mean slender, lightweight roots, while thick, robust stalks indicate a good root.

Green roots the size of a man's thumb or larger are considered good. Roots smaller than a man's little finger should not be dug. Of course, local growing conditions in some regions cause roots to grow short and stubby or long and slender, but the principle is still the same. Scrawny roots should not be harvested.

Root size is an issue that is currently making the rounds of regulatory agencies. The question is, should there be a minimum size for dried wild roots?

My thought on the subject is, yes. Still, I hope diggers will voluntarily practice size limitations so that further federal regulation of the ginseng trade is not required. If root size regulations were to take effect, they would likely stipulate that a buyer would not be able to purchase roots that contained more than a designated number of roots per pound. If small roots couldn't be sold, they presumably wouldn't be harvested.

The discussion will probably continue for several years before some decision is made on regulating root size. But now is the time for diggers to assess their digging practices and harvest only good-sized three- and four-prongers and leave the smaller three-prongers to grow larger and produce more seed. If all diggers stick to a code of digging only the largest plants, perhaps further regulation will not be needed.

In order to give diggers some guidance on root size and conservation, I have done an informal survey by grading several lots of dried roots from large to very small and counting the number of roots per pound in each grade. I will point out that grading roots by size is very subjective, and another grader may come up with somewhat different totals. Also, I did not have the luxury of counting tens of thousands of roots for a wide sampling. Still, I think you'll find the results to be representative and interesting.

AVERAGE NUMBER OF DRIED WILD ROOTS PER POUND BY SIZE

---

104 roots per pound—large
180 roots per pound—medium
276 roots per pound—small
378 roots per pound—very small

After counting roots, I set out to determine a voluntary conservation target range for ginseng harvest. This is an average harvest range that allows the digger to maximize his or her harvest in weight while curtailing the digging of immature roots. To do that, I simply determined the median point between large and medium roots (148 dried roots per pound), and the median point between medium and small roots (228 dried roots per pound).

As a result of this survey, I found my target conservation range to be 148 to 228 roots per pound, dried weight. To simplify matters I'm advocating a target range of 150 to 225 roots per pound. That is, the dried weight of the digger's harvest should fall within that range, or lower. Diggers who have more than 225 roots per pound in their lots are probably harvesting a lot of small roots.

For a number of years, my personal target range has been about 160 roots per pound. I pass over many small three-prongers, but I get top dollar for my roots and I find I am more efficient because

I'm not wasting time digging the small stuff. Remember, it takes just as long to dig a small root as it does to dig a large one. The time others waste on digging small roots I spend finding larger, more profitable roots. But realistically, nobody's going to get rich by digging wild ginseng no matter how he or she goes about it.

A friend of mine thought he had hit ginseng gold some years ago while working in the suburban Philadelphia area. He came across a woodlot that was carpeted with ginseng. He had never seen anything like it—thousands upon thousands of wild ginseng plants. Most people around Philadelphia had no idea what ginseng looks like, so the patch likely had been growing there since Ben Franklin's days. My friend informed the landowner and offered to show him how to dig and dry the ginseng if the owner would split the profits with him. The owner agreed. The two men spent the next few days digging ginseng and dreaming about early retirement. After all was said and done, the men split about twenty pounds of dried ginseng and pocketed $1,500 each—a nice sum for a week's work, but not exactly enough to retire on.

Nobody is going to get rich by digging wild ginseng. So be a conservationist, not an opportunist.

HAZARDS IN THE HUNT FOR WILD GINSENG

Ginseng terrain by its very nature can be rather intimidating to the tenderfoot outdoorsperson. Although you may stumble onto some ginseng in parklike settings close to civilization, my experience has been that the best patches of wild ginseng are located in difficult regions with precipitous hillsides, deep ravines, and complex switchback ridges. If you tackle such an area, you'll soon find that enthusiasm is no substitute for strong calf muscles—and a good topographic map. Know your limitations, both in physical conditioning and orienteering skills.

As in any woodland outing, a host of minor irritations can arise during the ginseng hunt. Biting and stinging insects may be encountered, so insect repellant and soothing lotions should be close at hand. Pulled muscles and minor strains can also occur.

A close encounter with a poisonous snake is another possibility in ginseng country, but it is not very likely. In all my years of hunting wild ginseng, I have only tangled with a rattlesnake once, when I nearly stepped on a four-and-a-half foot timber rattler slithering right at me. I emerged unscathed from the fray that ensued, but the showdown did end my enthusiasm for ginseng hunting, at least for the day! Copperheads are more numerous in my neck of the woods, but I have yet to come across one while hunting ginseng. Poisonous snakes generally fear humans and will give you a wide berth if you afford them the same consideration.

DIGGING, DRYING, AND MARKETING

Wild ginseng roots are harvested in the same manner as cultivated roots. Dig with care, because broken or damaged roots will bring a lower price. Also, avoid digging up smaller roots near the roots you wish to harvest. If you accidentally dig out an immature root, replant it immediately and firm the soil around it.

If you find a large root with a tendril running off the neck near the bud, you may be able to harvest the main root while leaving enough of the tendril to produce a plant again the following spring. Simply break the neck just beneath the tendril, leaving the bud and tendril in the ground while digging out the mature root. This is the only time you should break the neck of a ginseng root. If you have not disturbed the tendril too much, the bud may sprout during the next growing season. You can harvest the root and still have it produce a plant again the next year, although it will be much smaller.

Some diggers claim to have success with this method by breaking off and replanting the tendril and bud after completely unearthing the root, but I have found that exposing the tiny hair roots of the tendril usually kills the bud. Therefore, I carefully feel around the neck of each root as I dig and perform "surgery" as needed while the root is still in the ground.

On roots to be dried, snap the stem off where it joins the neck, but do not break any portion of the neck. The valuable neck will be long and somewhat fragile. It becomes more prone to breakage as it dries.

Wild roots are rinsed and dried in the same manner as woods-grown roots. Check in outdoor magazines and the Appendix for buyers of wild ginseng.

Some root buyers list different prices for different states, while others do not. The reason for the listings by state is simple: These buyers know from experience that roots from certain regions exhibit certain characteristics. They are able to pay more or less for certain types of roots, depending on the price they believe they will get after exporting the goods. Northern roots are considered to be the highest quality, but if you send in outstanding roots from more southerly states, you'll likely get close to the northern root price for your harvest.

How do you know you are getting top prices and accurate weighing from the dealer? I posed this question to Paul Hsu, a buyer of wild and cultivated ginseng. In his operation, wild roots get priority service. Each shipment is weighed and certified by two different people. Paul then personally inspects the shipment and grades it. Checks are cut within a few days and sent to the digger. My experience with other buyers has been similar.

Several ginseng vendors have also developed outlets for fresh wild ginseng roots. I've never sold fresh roots, but it would save the digger the hassle of drying roots. If you would like to sell your wild or wild-simulated roots fresh, check with the buyers listed in the Appendix. Be aware that only a few dealers in the United States handle fresh roots, as the market for them is limited.

Chapter 8

Ginseng and Traditional Herbal Medicine

Ginseng is a tonic to the five viscera, quieting the spirits, establishing the soul, allaying fear, expelling evil effluvia, brightening the eye, opening the heart, benefitting the understanding and, if taken for some time, it will invigorate the body and prolong life.

The first known account of ginseng usage, recorded approximately five thousand years ago by Chinese Emperor Shen Nung

The origin of all ancient drugs was herbs, in both Eastern and Western medicine. Their use and classification evolved very differently in each culture, however. Western herbalists placed herbs in proper scientific families according to physical attributes. Conversely, Eastern practitioners classified herbs according to their effects on the human body. The concept that "all medicine is food" also developed in the Chinese tradition. Because of this, ginseng became the most highly prized medicinal agent in Chinese herbal medicine, while in the West it was inventoried as little more than a glorified parsnip (another Araliaceae).

Now the influence of traditional Chinese medicine has spread around the globe. Listings for acupuncture specialists, for example, can be found in phone books across the United States, and Chinese herbs are commonplace in American natural food stores.

The ginseng root contains a variety of complex constituents, perhaps the most of any medicinal plant known to man. Researchers have found in ginseng monosaccharides, disaccharides, trisaccharides, polysaccharides, amino acids, peptides, proteins, alkaloids, lipids, fatty acids, phytosterols, ginseng oils, organic acids, polyacetylenes, flavonoids, and terpenes. The major active components in ginseng roots, however, are saponins called ginsenosides or panaxisides.

Ginsenosides are sugars that constitute about 3 to 6 percent of the dried root weight and are the substances that cause a slight foaming when ginseng tea is brewed. There are about thirteen main ginsenosides, but in wild ginseng up to twenty-three ginsenosides can be found, most of them in trace amounts. In cultivated ginseng, researchers can usually identify ten or eleven ginsenosides.

Individual ginsenosides are classified and given an R value alphabetically in increasing order—Ra, Rb1, Rb2, and so on. The two main groupings of ginsenosides are Rb and Rg. Rg ginsenosides are stimulants and are found in much higher quantities in Asiatic ginseng than in the American variety. At least two thirds of the Asian ginsenosides are Rg1 and Rg2; in American ginseng less than one third are Rg. Therefore, Asiatic ginseng is much more stimulating that ours. American ginseng is high in Rb, Rc, Rd, and Re. These are all relaxants, so American ginseng is considered to be more calming.

Curiously, ginsenosides taken singularly as drugs react strangely and may even be detrimental to one's health, but when they are used together, they can be beneficial. Western pharmacology would prescribe either an Rb stimulant or an Rg relaxant, but never both in combination. In contrast, herbal formulas are employed as a whole and are rarely used singularly. Four to ten herbs might be used to treat a disease. Some would absorb toxicity, some would enhance energy, and some would strengthen bodily functions. Traditional herbal formulas are used to treat a patient as a total person with many interrelated aspects. The aim of this approach is to "balance the body" while neutralizing all aspects of the disease.

The idea of balance, not only in the body but throughout the universe, has evolved over many centuries. Early Chinese Taoists theorized that there was an omnipotent force in the universe, called *chi*. They believed that the power of *chi* was ceaseless, moving endlessly between positive and negative forces. This constant but balanced interaction between opposing natural forces, yin and yang, was thought to be the basis for existence throughout the universe.

The modern Chinese also regard *chi* as the life force, and they classify the body system into yin and yang. Yin represents the negative, dark, cold, and feminine. Yang is positive, light, warm, and masculine. All ginseng is considered yang food, but Asian ginseng is considered more yang. On a continuum with total yin as 0 and total yang as 100, for example, American ginseng might be considered a 55 while Asian ginseng may be 75 or 80. Therefore, each ginseng is used under different circumstances to achieve balance in the system and to maintain *chi,* the essence of life.

A celebrated influence on ginseng's ancient reputation as a

panacea, or all-healing medicine, was the Doctrine of Signatures. This ideology, developed on the European, North American, and Asian continents, suggested that a plant resembling a human part could be used to treat an illness in that part. Since the strange little ginseng roots often resembled the entire human body, they were revered by various cultures as a medicinal agent capable of treating all bodily ailments and increasing fertility.

There are three classifications of Chinese medicines—mild, moderate, and curative. A mild medicine has no long-term harmful effect and acts as a tonic. Moderate medicine is stronger, perhaps having both tonic and curative effects. The long-term use of a moderate medicine could be harmful, since the curative portion would be a toxin meant to destroy some specific illness in the body. Curative medicines are toxic, can be harmful in long-term usage, and must be carefully monitored by a physician. Most Western medicines are curative.

Ginseng is listed as a mild medicine in Shen Nung's *Pen Ts'ao* (500 A.D. edition). It is not harmful for long-term usage and its effects are enumerated as follows:

- Ginseng strengthens the internal organs.
- Ginseng has a tranquilizing effect.
- Ginseng prevents headache, fatigue, and exhaustion.
- Ginseng increases resistance to disease.
- Ginseng improves vision.
- Ginseng improves mental capacity.
- Ginseng strengthens general well-being and prolongs life.

More recent medical reports from China claim that ginseng also facilitates the formation of red blood cells, aids in the treatment of diabetes, normalizes pulmonary functions, and detoxifies poisons. Other accounts indicate that ginseng encourages cell repair after exposure to radiation (such as cancer treatments), relieves symptoms of menopause, and improves sexual behavior in animals. There is even a claim that hens lay more eggs after they eat ginseng.

Western researchers generally cast a suspicious eye on ginseng research, believing that the data are far from adequate. They cite the lack of double-blind crossover experiments, which reduce the bias and placebo effects, and point out that frequently too few subjects are involved in testing to get accurate statistical data. Experiments are also compromised when ginseng of unknown composition is used, and unfavorable data are rarely reported. The fact that ginseng research is usually paid for by ginseng trade associations has not been lost on investigators, who often are unable to duplicate published results during independent testing. Nonetheless, Western medical researchers have admitted that ginsenosides do have certain in vitro activities. Until the significance of these effects on humans are proved or disproved, ginseng is likely to remain a medical enigma in the minds of most Westerners.

In the United States, ginseng—both American and Asian—is perhaps best known as a general tonic rather than as a medicine, but the English word *tonic* doesn't really do justice to the Chinese concept of *bou*. *Tonic* has the connotation of "snake oil"—a concoction without real medicinal value—while *bou* means balancing, assisting, mending, repairing, enhancing, and replacing. A tonic medicine might be a more accurate description of ginseng as Easterners see it.

The word *adaptogen* has also been used to describe ginseng's ability to increase the body's nonspecific resistance to physical and mental stress—the ability to bounce back to normal. *Adaptogen* was coined by a Russian researcher in the late 1950s and ginseng was frequently used in the Russian cosmonaut program because of its adaptogen qualities. Interestingly, Asians often refer to ginseng as a normalizer. Since American ginseng is the more relaxing ginseng, it has been long recognized as the best normalizer for people of Western descent, reputed in the East for having hot temperaments.

Ginseng is generally prescribed by herbal practitioners to be taken over a long period of time, much like a daily vitamin tablet. It is not a drug to be used only when the body is suffering some ill effect, although it is sometimes used this way.

It's unfortunate that ginseng's historical reputation as an all-healing medicine has been rather coarsely reduced to "cure-all" in our trend-loving society. Perhaps we should stand back, forget about the Western concept of a single chemical having a single effect, and try to grasp the time-honored applications of ginseng in the cultures of India, Russia, China, Korea, Japan, and Native America. Can the teeming millions who used ginseng over thousands of years have been so wrong? Would a modern Chinese peasant really pay half a year's salary for a pound of wild American ginseng if it were unlikely to provide the desired results? Has ginseng been rejected by Western medicine, not because it is ineffective, but because it does not fit neatly into the system?

GINSENG USES

Hundreds of claims have been made for ginseng usage, and many of them may be valid. Nevertheless, I can make no medical affirmations, direct or implied, and would certainly advise that a doctor be consulted for the treatment of any ailment. It is generally accepted that ginseng can be taken in addition to other drugs without risk of incompatibility, although a physician should always be told that a patient is taking or intends to take ginseng while undergoing a course of prescribed medicine. With that in mind, here are a few of the reported actions of ginseng.

Gastrointestinal Ailments

Ginseng is thought to offer general relaxation to the gastrointestinal system. Some experimental data indicate that ginseng can prevent the release of very acidic gastric juices, therefore reducing stomach irritation while promoting digestion and elimination. Many claims have been made that ginseng is helpful in treating ulcers, upset stomachs, and constipation. Interestingly, the use of ginseng as a stomach remedy was one of the earliest-known medicinal applications of the root in Native American culture.

Alcohol Detoxification

Ginseng prompts the liver to expel poisons quickly, and since alcohol is a poison, ginseng tends to reduce intoxication by clearing it from the liver. Clinical experiments have shown that a person taking ginseng while drinking an alcoholic beverage will have lower blood alcohol levels than a person drinking the same beverage without also consuming ginseng. Because of this effect, ginseng slices are often served in Korean restaurants when alcoholic beverages are offered. Some people also claim that ginseng is a good antidote for a hangover.

Blood Pressure and Cholesterol

Ginseng appears to have some influence in normalizing blood pressure, whether it be high or low. The biological reason for this is not completely understood, but ginseng may restore blood pressure to normal levels by correcting some imbalance in the system. In clinical trials with patients suffering from high blood pressure, ginseng was shown to produce a small but consistent reduction in blood pressure. Cholesterol levels have also normalized after the daily ingestion of ginseng for several months, with patients showing a reduction in overall cholesterol and an increase in the beneficial HDL cholesterol.

Diabetes

In laboratory trials with diabetic rats, ginseng reduced blood sugar levels and doubled the average lifespan of the animals. A Chinese study on humans showed that a diet regimen incorporating ginseng resulted in reduced insulin requirements for the patients. Subjective symptoms such as fatigue were also reduced. Conversely, ginseng also appears to raise blood glucose levels when they fall dangerously low. In animal tests, ginseng supplements have counteracted hypoglycemia induced by the administration of excess insulin. Ginseng apparently helps normalize blood glucose levels, whether they be high or low.

Sexual Potency

One of the most fabled powers of ginseng is its aphrodisiac effect. It is now thought that ginseng helps restore sexual function by increasing general vitality rather than increasing virility. Some studies, however, have shown a hormonal connection between ginseng and human reproduction potential. One human study indicated that, after taking ginseng, patients suffering from a numerical deficiency in sperm had higher sperm counts. In animal tests, rats ingesting ginseng developed larger ovaries than the control animals. Ginseng also encouraged the development of sex organs in young mice and stimulated them to reach puberty faster than untreated mice. Because of this possible hormonal influence on reproductive systems, *children should not take ginseng prior to reaching puberty.*

Stress and Endurance

Regular use of ginseng may help the body cope with stress. Ginsenosides seem to stimulate the body to increase overall resistance, thereby helping a person to both cope better with stress and to return to normal activity more quickly after being stressed. Chinese soldiers traditionally consume ginseng on the battlefield for the purpose of resisting stress and shock. Animal experiments have shown that rats fed Asian ginseng recovered more quickly from cold or heat stress than did a control group. In other tests, rats fed ginseng were able to swim up to 50 percent longer than rats not receiving ginseng. In a rather bizarre Russian experiment during which rats were allowed to swim until death, rats fed ginseng survived approximately an hour longer than a control group.

A human test involving nurses changing from day to night duty showed that those taking ginseng performed better on tests of mood, competence, and general performance than did nurses not taking ginseng.

Longevity

One of the earliest uses of ginseng was to prolong life. Mindful that the mere extension of life into old age was of little value, the ancient Chinese found meaning in extending a healthy existence. Ginseng was the medicine of choice for this gerontological effect. Today, Chinese research indicates that ginseng retards the degeneration of cells, acts as an antioxidant, and improves general health, thus delaying the aging process and promoting longevity. Additional European studies indicate that ginseng usage by the elderly leads to an improvement in mood, concentration, alertness, memory, and problem-solving ability.

GINSENG PRODUCTS

Ginseng roots are made into a variety of products—extracts and elixirs, powders, tablets, capsules, tea, soft drinks, chewing gum, and cosmetics. Before being manufactured into consumer products, ginseng is treated in one of two ways to produce either red or white ginseng, with red being the more valuable type.

To produce red ginseng, natural white roots are steamed so that they take on a translucent reddish-brown color and a unique bittersweet flavor. The process of steaming and sun drying for long-term preservation goes back about one thousand years and is mainly practiced in the Orient.

Only the best roots are chosen for red ginseng. They are

steamed for about three hours in secret ingredients, with the brew specifically calibrated for the geographic origin of the roots. The next step is sun drying for about fifteen days. Automated dryers are used in inclement weather. After drying, the roots are trimmed, packaged, and vacuum sealed. These premium red ginseng roots can be chewed, soaked in an alcoholic beverage to form an elixir or in hot water to make an extract, or ground into powder for tea and capsules. The extract is sometimes concentrated into a thick brown paste and encapsulated.

White ginseng products are processed from ginseng roots that are dried but not steamed. American ginseng is nearly always processed as white ginseng. The Koreans sometimes peel the skin from their white roots before packaging. White ginseng can be used in the same manner as red ginseng.

As a pleasant daily rejuvenator, ginseng is usually consumed in a tea. Ginseng roots can be sliced or ground and added to hot water, but never in a metal container. Ginseng teas are steeped a few minutes longer than other teas so that all the ginsenosides can be extracted into the drink. Other teas can be mixed with ginseng tea in order to mute its somewhat bitter taste, although the recognized Asian practice is to take ginseng tea alone. Traditionally, two consecutive cups of tea are made with the same root slices in order to extract all the ginsenosides.

Father Pierre Jartoux reported the customary Chinese method of preparation in the early 1700s:

> The root is to be cut into thin slices, and put into an earthen pot well glazed, and filled with about a quarter of a pint of water Paris measure. The pot must be well covered and set to boil over a gentle fire, and when the water is consumed to the quantity of a cupful, a little sugar is to be mixed with it, and it is to be drunk immediately. After

this, as much more water is to be put into the pot upon the remainder, and to be boiled as before, to extract all the juice and what remains of the spirituous part of the root. These two doses are to be taken, one in the morning and the other at night.

Ginseng capsules are quite popular in the United States. The ginseng dosage recommended by most herbalists is one or two five hundred-milligram capsules of ginseng per day, swallowed or in a tea. Ginseng is considered nontoxic, but like anything, it should be taken in moderation.

An elixir (or tincture) of American ginseng can be concocted by placing a whole ginseng root (or roots) in an alcoholic beverage such as gin or rum. The bottle is left standing for several weeks, during which time the ginsenosides infuse the liquid. The beverage is then ready to drink. In the Appalachians, an elixir of white lightnin' and ginseng has been known to appear on medicine shelves from time to time.

Chapter 9

Ginseng Questions and Answers

We entered a vale at 5 o'clock, then crossed a run and rode along a rich level for several miles, and under the delightful protection of very tall trees that brought us to a creek, a branch of the Susquehanah, where we lodged surrounded by ginseng.

John Bartram,
in his *Travels from Pensilvania
to Onondago, Oswego, and
Lake Ontario in Canada,*
London, 1751

Following are some of the questions I have been asked over the years by prospective ginseng cultivators and diggers. The question and answer format is meant to present straightforward information about ginseng and allow me to offer some personal observations along the way.

HOW LONG HAVE YOU BEEN INVOLVED WITH GINSENG?

About thirty years. Today I live along the Susquehanna River in Lancaster County, Pennsylvania, where wild ginseng is rare. However, as a youngster in Fayette County, Pennsylvania, I dug wild roots and sold them locally at the general store. We called ginseng "jing-sang"; I was shocked when I found out how it was really spelled. I remember the excitement in the mountains when the price hit thirty dollars per pound for wild ginseng. That was quite some time ago. It was only natural that I attempted to cultivate ginseng, mainly out of curiosity. Over the years I have tried small-plot cultivation under both artificial and natural shade. Everything was trial and error.

My first artificial shade garden was under wood lathe. It was very small, maybe eight by sixteen feet. I just dug up part of my parent's yard, erected some shade, and transplanted ginseng from the wild. No soil test, no fertilizer, no nothing. It grew like crazy! Looking back, I see how remarkable it was that I got any yield at all, since I didn't use pesticides. Of course, my mother wasn't too happy about having what she called an Indian burial ground in the backyard, so after a year or two it came down. One thing I've discovered over the years is that you don't need a big parcel of shaded land to grow ginseng. When I lived in town, I had a couple dozen plants growing under my deck. It was a great marketing feature when I sold the house. The first people who looked at my home wanted to buy it—as long as I left the ginseng for them!

Right now, I have ginseng plants tucked between my shed and a hedgerow, and underneath some shrubbery. I also have a woodland garden a few miles away, but I really enjoy having some plants near the house.

WHAT TYPE OF HABITAT DO YOU LOOK FOR WHEN HUNTING WILD GINSENG?

I've hunted wild ginseng in Pennsylvania, West Virginia, Maryland, and Tennessee, and good habitat is remarkably similar everywhere. Maple, beech, and hickory with some tulip poplar mixed in is the best habitat. I don't like an area where oak is the predominate species. Oak tends to like a very sour soil, which I don't think ginseng tolerates well. Some oak mixed with maple and poplar is fine. I stay away from boggy areas and dry ridge tops. The rich, mellow soil of rolling hardwood benches and ravines is where you'll find wild ginseng.

Good weeds are the best indicators of favorable ginseng habitat. Hardwood forests are a blend of many micro-environments, and forest floor conditions change repeatedly across any tract. Not every section of a forest is suitable for ginseng, so look for companion plants before beginning a search for ginseng. Good weeds don't necessarily have ginseng nearby—that would make it too easy—but ginseng usually has a few good weeds around it. A quick scan of a woodland tract for good weeds can quickly tell you whether or not conditions are right for ginseng. Some good weeds will tolerate sunlight better than ginseng, so only use good weeds as an indication of soil quality and not shade quality.

HOW DO YOU PLANT YOUR GINSENG GARDEN?

For sizeable plots, or high-intensity cultivation, I use broadcast seeding—simply strolling through the garden and casting seed by hand. This method does tend to bunch the plants, however, so I mix sand with the seed in order to provide better dispersion. The sand grains replace some of the seeds in each handful, thereby reducing the number of seeds in each cast. This is an easy way to obtain good spacing when broadcasting seeds.

After broadcasting, the soil can be raked and mulched, or simply covered with several inches of loose mulch, which will slowly compact over the seeds. I use wheat straw because it is readily available in farm country, but just about any type of organic mulch can be used. The only type I would not use is pine needles. They just don't feel right to me. Realistically, mulch might not even be required if your seeds are planted and covered with about ½ to ¾ inch of soil. One of my nicest beds has no mulch at all. It's just bare dirt. And I'm gathering sixty to eighty seeds from each two-foot-high, six-year-old plant.

On small plots, I prefer to plant with a seeder. Nearly any type of commercial seeder will do the trick if you can get the right hole size for ginseng's odd-shaped seeds. Or, forget the seeder and drop seeds into a furrow by hand. It takes a little longer, but I find it to be both accurate and a labor of love. Right now, I'm planting every eight inches in rows about eight inches apart for eight-by-eight-inch spacing. With sixteen-inch paths running lengthwise at six-foot intervals, this spacing method requires only thirteen pounds of seeds per acre.

WHAT ABOUT WILD-SIMULATED PLANTINGS?

The most realistic approach to true wild-simulated "cultivation" is to simply walk through your woodland planting seeds here and there in rich fertile soil. Small, widely scattered patches will require little maintenance. If you like, you can just plant seeds and forget about them for ten years. From a personal viewpoint, modest attention in the way of an occasional pesticide application is beneficial and will not lower the value of the roots.

DO VETERAN GINSENG
DIGGERS HAVE AN ADVANTAGE
IN GROWING WILD-SIMULATED GINSENG?

I don't think there's any real advantage, as long as the novice cultivators do their homework. Veteran 'sangers may have a slight edge in spotting good habitat, but they don't necessarily use that to their advantage. I knew a digger who transplanted a number of wild plants to a poor location and then complained about how little growth he got over the years. When I told him it didn't look like a good site to me, he said it was the best spot he could think of—to keep other diggers from finding his 'sang! Most 'sangers are so secretive that they consider concealment as the top priority and don't plant in the best areas. After all, that's where other diggers are likely to come poking around. Novices who plant on a good tract and keep an eye on their ginseng will be farther ahead than 'sangers who intentionally conceal their plants in a poor location.

DO FEDERAL FOOD-PROCESSING
REGULATIONS APPLY TO GINSENG?

Ginseng is considered a raw agricultural commodity (RAC) and is therefore subject to pesticide residue restrictions. Recent studies have shown that pesticide residues from dried ginseng samples are within the range considered safe for other food commodities.

There is currently some concern in the ginseng industry about stricter interpretation of the Delaney Clause, a 1958 federal law that allows no trace of a cancer-causing substance that might concentrate in processed food. Until recently, the Environmental Protection Agency had viewed the Delaney Clause as negligible-risk rather than zero-tolerance legislation because scientific advances since 1958 have made it possible to find minuscule amounts of a substance in food. A 1992 court ruling has forced the Environmental Protection Agency to follow the law's zero-risk standard—but only in processed foods. Raw foods are subject to a more lenient risk-benefit standard for pesticide residues.

The problem facing the ginseng industry is that the Environmental Protection Agency has not yet determined whether fresh or dried ginseng is the raw agricultural commodity. Breakdown residue from Dithane DF (mancozeb, a maneb fungicide) has been found in ginseng roots. This residue, ETU, is a known carcinogen that has been shown to be within the negligible-risk guidelines in dried ginseng roots. However, if fresh ginseng roots (instead of dried roots) are determined to be the RAC, ETU will be considered a food additive when the roots are dried, and there will be a zero-tolerance level. In this case, Dithane DF will not be available for use in ginseng production.

The loss of Dithane DF for ginseng production would likely lead to a major decline of the industry in the United States. The only alternative to mancozeb is a combination of Rovral 50W/Kocide DF and Aliette WDG at ten times the cost per application. And these pesticides are not as effective as Dithane DF in controlling Alternaria blight.

The other alternative is for the Environmental Protection Agency to view dried ginseng as the RAC. If this determination is made, the negligible-risk standard applies and Dithane DF will be available for use on ginseng.

The Delaney Clause creates great confusion in the food-processing industry, and the National Academy of Sciences has recommended changing the law to a negligible-risk standard. Consumer groups, on the other hand, want the Delaney Clause expanded to include raw foods in the zero-tolerance standard.

Whatever the outcome of the Delaney Clause debate, food-processing regulations will change, and the Environmental Protection Agency could offer a ruling on ginseng at any time. The decision may or may not alter the list of chemicals approved for use on ginseng. You can see how important it is for the ginseng cultivator to stay up-to-date on the status of all chemical controls used in the ginseng garden.

IS AMERICAN GINSENG CULTIVATED
ANYWHERE OUTSIDE THE UNITED STATES?

Canada is a major player in the cultivated American ginseng market. Of course, portions of Canada are within the historic range of American ginseng, so it's only natural that cultivation would occur there. The Canadians have successfully expanded ginseng cultivation into British Columbia and are subsidizing ginseng farms in that region.

I do not know of any large-scale ginseng cultivation in Europe, but it has been tried on a limited scale in several European countries. Some attempts have been made at cultivation in South America, and a growing number of entrepreneurs in Australia are quite excited about the potential profit in raising ginseng. Interestingly, during my recent visit to a ginseng farm in Wisconsin, an Aussie dropped in to gather information about cultivation. The Australians are pursuing ginseng cultivation in their country for two reasons. They currently import quite a bit of ginseng for use in natural remedies and pharmaceuticals. They would like to grow their own ginseng to supply this local demand. Also, geographically they are considerably closer to the Asian consumers than are American growers. They would eventually like to develop a thriving ginseng business on their continent and undercut American prices. Realistically, the Aussies face major problems in soil types and climatic conditions. Not the least of their obstacles is that they are located in the southern hemisphere, where the seasons are exactly opposite of ours. Their winter is our summer and vice versa, so the seeds they purchase from American growers sprout six months out of sync! Some growers have apparently overcome these hurdles, but it remains to be seen whether Australian ginseng farming will ever be profitable enough to challenge the North American market.

In China, American ginseng has been planted from seed sold by U.S. and Canadian growers. You can see how eager the Asians are to have our native ginseng. If American ginseng becomes well established in the Orient, it will mount a major challenge to American roots cultivated under artificial shade. It seems somewhat short-sighted of North American growers to sell our precious American seed overseas, but it was probably inevitable in the current global economy.

WHAT ARE YOUR PREDICTIONS FOR THE FUTURE OF AMERICAN GINSENG?

The market for American ginseng is going to grow, particularly the markets for woodsgrown and wild-simulated roots. Wild ginseng is becoming rare and expensive. Wild-simulated will take the place of wild in the future. In fact, a lot of the wild that is being sold now is realistically wild-simulated. Diggers are harvesting ginseng that they planted in earlier years, so it's not truly wild ginseng. The size is getting smaller; roots are getting younger. Keep in mind that the wild ginseng harvest will probably never increase. I feel certain that some wild-simulated ginseng is being certified as wild, so the true wild ginseng harvest is even lower than the statistics indicate.

Landowners who have an idle woodlot can put it to work as a retirement account. I'd definitely recommend woodsgrown and wild-simulated cultivation. Ninety-nine percent of the ginseng farms outside the natural range of American ginseng use artificial shade. No matter what happens to the lower quality artificial-shade roots, our woodsgrown and wild-simulated roots will remain strong in the world market.

Chapter 10

A Field Trip in Search of the Wild Root

In passing over the Mountains, I met numbers of Persons & Pack horses going in with Ginsang & for salt and other articles at the Markets below.

George Washington,
Laurel Mountains of
Fayette County, Pennsylvania,
12 September 1784

It is September 12, 1994. I am hunting ginseng in the Laurel Mountains mentioned by Washington in his diary, perhaps even standing on the same ridge where he met the colonial 'sangers 210 years before. This is the story of my journey and my reflections.

I stop near the top of the ridge and wipe a trickle of sweat from my forehead. The humidity climbs quickly with the mid-morning sun, its sultry embrace pressing the flesh with insistence if not form. A colossal maple near the pinnacle suddenly whispers a soft song of relief as an errant breeze beckons in the treetops. But on the ground the air is still, and in a moment even the loftiest leaves cease their seductive dance.

My dirt-streaked hand feels for the ginseng root in my belt pack. There are several gnarled roots in the pack, but only one is *the* root. I pull out a grandaddy of two ounces or so and run a finger softly along the twisted neck scars, counting silently. I stop at thirty-eight. Forty years ago this magnificent ginseng root was an unformed embryo inside a pale seed within a crimson berry. Somehow it had found its way to a spot of dark, virgin soil, eluding chipmunks and mice for its two-year germination period while the tiny embryo inside swelled until the shell cracked open. I can see the Lilliputian beginnings of the man-root in my mind, a sliver of ivory on a golden nugget, the robust life force within impelling it toward the center of the earth while its tiny tri-leaf crown climbed incessantly toward the light on some handsome spring day. I question how the plant had escaped the fires and the logging operations that ravaged the region, and how many ginseng diggers had slipped across this ridge without noticing its dark green foliage or the brilliant scarlet of its berries. I wonder how many of the plant's progeny now inhabit the surrounding slopes and ravines.

My thoughts digress further, to a time when the native people of the continent ruled the western boundaries of Penn's Woods. It was here that the Cherokee and the Mohawks met, sometimes violently, as Cherokee hunters pushed north from the Carolinas while scouting parties from the Iroquois Six Nations moved south into the Appalachians, exploring, hunting, conquering.

For the Anglos on the North American continent, Pennsylvania's Laurel Mountains were a paradox of wonder and horror 250 years ago. In 1754, a young lieutenant colonel in the Virginia Militia named George Washington wrote of a "charming field for an encounter" as he moved along the Braddock Trail a few ridges to my west. Soon after that log entry, Washington was to hastily construct Fort Necessity and suffer his first military defeat at the hands of French and Indian allies in the Great Meadows of southwestern Pennsylvania. The opening volley of the French and Indian War had been fired a few days before that, no more than a long cannonshot across the mountains from where I now stand. Those two engagements opened the bloodiest conflict of the eighteenth century, a conflict destined to last seven years, wrest control of the Appalachians from the French, spread across three continents, and change the course of world history.

Daniel Boone likely passed this way as he crossed into the heart of American ginseng country to settle Boonesboro, Kentucky. I reflect on the next war to be fought for control of this region, the Revolutionary War, and Colonel Boone's capture at the hands of Native Americans acting under British orders. His escape and grueling 160-mile journey in four days to defend his Kentucky namesake against a prolonged Indian attack are the stuff of legends.

My thoughts begin to run wild. I imagine that Dan'l crept around this very knob just a few lucky steps ahead of an Indian war party, and before that, perhaps George Washington marched across this mountain under the watchful eyes of the native inhabitants he had been sent to fight.

A cold shiver grips my spine and the warmth of the day suddenly goes unnoticed. I decide to move quickly around the point ahead. Eyes darting and ears straining, I do my best Indian imitation, stepping quickly but cautiously through the leaf litter. The gurgle of an unnamed run in a no-name hollow fades away as I move into a high cove, striding to the beat of war drums in my mind and the lonely wail of a red-tailed hawk above. After a few moments I step onto a lofty bluff adorned with ginseng and stand still with time in the remote reaches of Appalachia.

The unmuffled roar of an ancient farm truck snaps me back to the present. A faint wisp of blue engine smoke rising from the valley below leaves no doubt that George Washington, Daniel Boone, and all the Native Americans are long gone from this place. But wild ginseng, the mystical plant of the Chinese dynasties, is alive and well in the Appalachian Mountains.

Today, I am hunting ginseng on the same hills crossed by colonists centuries before. It was Indian country then, rugged and hostile. Even now it remains much the same: rough terrain, steep mountains, and countless ravines opening to deep, unspoiled valleys—ginseng country.

My eyes sweep once more across the highlands that reach out and touch the sky on a distant velvet line, then turn to the patch of ginseng that surrounds my feet. It takes me a few minutes to mine the four-prongers from the rocky earth and plant the precious berries nearby. Then I contemplate whether to dig the three-prongers. I like to leave some seed producers in each patch, so I decide to harvest only the largest three-pronger. The others will remain to carry on the legacy of wild American ginseng.

But this tenacious plant stymies me. My digging trowel clanks against stone and, try as I might, I cannot extract the root from a narrow rock fissure. I can see the man-root wedged securely in its stony abode, but I cannot possess it. With a tip of my hat to the victor, I slip the trowel into my back pocket and push seeds from the plant's crimson berries into other rock crevices. With any luck these seeds will also grow to maturity, safely tucked away from a digger's trowel, disseminating still more seeds across the Appalachians.

A hint of scarlet on a lower slope catches my eye and I slide down to it quickly. It turns out to be the berries of an Indian turnip. This is a good weed, a companion plant, so I cast about looking for ginseng nearby. I find none. The terrain looks favorable, however, with splendid woodsy soil and high, filtered shade. I reach into my pack for a bag of seeds from my cultivated plants. A few strokes with my trowel open several furrows in the good earth, and I drop a handful of seeds and cover them quickly.

I like to supplement the wild ginseng population by planting additional seeds from my garden as I walk across the mountains. The trick to making this work is to plant near good companion plants such as black cohosh and Indian turnip. I call these plants "nature's pH meters," as they indicate that soil conditions are right for ginseng. Planting ginseng seeds near companion plants ensures future good hunting for forest gold.

Heading down again, the good weeds fade away and my prospects for ginseng dim. My eye catches an unexpected glint of silver against green moss, however, and I soon kneel beside a partially hidden spring. Reflections disintegrate as I splash a handful of the cool liquid onto my face. With a shake of my head, I fling a misty spray against a moss-covered boulder at the head of the spring. Here, a radiant beam of sunlight pierces the shadows, and I look up to see water droplets sparkling like rhinestones on the rock's luxurious emerald coat.

A bit of rusty metal hidden beneath humus near the boulder catches my interest. I pull the weathered barrel band loose, scattering dirt haphazardly into the clear springwater. A few quick strokes with my digger on the rocky rim of the spring-branch turn up shards of crockware, a broken mason jar, and a tiny, twisted piece of copper tubing. Now I search in earnest for the remnants of a moonshine still that must have stood on this spot many years before.

Western Pennsylvania has always been moonshine country. The three-year Whiskey Rebellion from 1791 to 1794 was centered around the Scotch-Irish farmers of this region who had precious little to their name other than their land and their crops. Making whiskey was a way to sell excess grain each year since it was lighter—and a lot more profitable—than rye or corn in transport. When the new Congress of the United States passed an excise tax on whiskey in order to pay debts incurred during the Revolutionary War, the pioneer-farmers were furious. In their minds, they had just fought a war to be free from excise taxes and they weren't about to go back to such aristocratic rulings. The result was the first civil war of this country, a revolt by force of arms that prompted an incensed President Washington to write, "The west is balanced as if on the edge of a feather . . . and could fall either way." President Washington himself led troops to put down the Whiskey Rebellion and so went down in the annals of American history as the only commander in chief to lead soldiers into battle.

I search around the spring for remnants of the rough-hewn building that most certainly would have stood nearby, but I come up empty handed. The years have erased nearly every sign of man's former presence here. I decide to sit for a moment near the cool spring and reflect on another ancient moonshine still that operated halfway across the county a full century before.

The Bill Pritts Distillery was the most famous still in Saltlick Township, Fayette County, circa 1900. Bill Pritts was an ornery man with a spitfire of a wife and a smattering of pioneer spirit left over from the Whiskey Rebellion. He was bold enough to stick his picture on jugs of illegal liquor, so he naturally drew quite a bit of attention from the local constabulary and federal "revennoers." Records from the period indicate that an eight-year search for the able-bodied mountaineer, from 1892 to 1900, finally met with success in finding his hideout. The officers who crept up on the cabin got more than they bargained for, however, when the family dog, said to be just as ornery as his owner, let loose with a howl and Bill's high-spirited wife, Hannah, sallied forth to do battle, armed with her broom. The agents quickly abandoned the fight, retreated down the mountain, and eventually outran the woman and the dog, although the dog carried the chase a good mile farther than Mrs. Pritts according to local gospel.

Bill Pritts was eventually captured—while taking a nap in the woods as the story goes—and led away in handcuffs. Remarked one of the federal marshals involved in his capture, "Remember, the game of hide and seek with U.S. Marshals is against heavy odds and detracts from the pleasures of life."

Since he was considered more of a hero than a culprit in western Pennsylvania, Bill was set free with the understanding that if he made any more liquor, he'd pay the appropriate tax.

My ninetysomething great aunt still tattles about the hoedowns held at the "still-house" during her youth. It was a time of magnificent fun for all, particularly for Bill and Hannah, who loved to kick up their heels, even into old age.

As I stand and brush off the seat of my pants, I notice a few small two-prongers tucked near a fallen log. These are not legal game in Pennsylvania, since state law restricts ginseng harvest to plants with three or more prongs. My hand goes into my pack again, this time drawing out a small bag of garden fertilizer. Over the past few years, I've started fertilizing immature ginseng plants in the wild. Some old-time diggers will likely cringe at the thought of fertilizing wild ginseng, but what's the harm in helping wild ginseng along a little? I sprinkle a handful of fertilizer around the small plants and work it into the ground with my finger. It takes only a couple of seconds and should produce bigger plants with berries in the following year.

As I tuck the fertilizer away, I eye the ground in hopes of finding a dried and withered ginseng stalk sticking up from the leaves on the forest floor. Something tells me there's a parent plant tucked away nearby, an old bull root that hasn't sent up a plant this year. In a few seconds I find it, a withered stalk almost unnoticeable against the mosaic pattern of fallen leaves. My breath comes quicker as I dig, fingers from one hand following the long neck while the other hand works the trowel. I can tell the root is massive, perhaps even bigger than the largest in my sack. I brush the soil away carefully and find a bonus—a small tendril running off the neck near the bud. I quickly break the neck just below it. The main root comes free in my hand while a small portion of the neck with bud and tendril remains in the soil. This bud will sprout the next spring and produce another ginseng plant if I have left enough of the root tendril undisturbed. By doing this, I can harvest the root while leaving a portion of it to sprout and propagate again.

Now the sun stands high in the sky and it is time for me to return to the modern world. I leave the pulse of the Appalachians behind as I stroll down the hollow, still reminiscing about the resourceful people who have held stewardship over the ginseng on this mountain throughout the centuries. Near my journey's end a cascading waterfall fills the air with mist and music, and I think about the destiny of the ginseng roots in my sack—of their journey across a great ocean to the hustle and bustle of the Orient and eventually, I hope, into the hands of a common man like myself.

I wish him well.

Appendix

SEED AND ROOTLET SUPPLIERS

Buckhorn Ginseng
Route 4
Richland Center, WI 53581

Hare Farms, Inc.
RR 1
Waterford, Ontario
Canada NOE 1Y0

Hsu's Ginseng Enterprises
T6819 County Highway W
P.O. Box 509
Wausau, WI 54402-0509

Ohio River Ginseng
and Fur, Inc.
P.O. Box 2347
Route 267
East Liverpool, OH 43920

Pickerell's Ginseng Farm
258 Ennis Mill Road
Hodgenville, KY 42748

Roots O Gold
Box 92
Le Center, MN 56057

GINGENG ROOT PURCHASERS

Buckhorn Ginseng
Route 4
Richland Center, WI 53581

Chap Hing Cheung
Canada Ltd.
104 Lynngate Place
London, Ontario
Canada N6K 1S5

Hershey International, Inc.
8210 Carlisle Pike
York Springs, PA 17372

Hsu's Ginseng Enterprises, Inc.
T6819 County Highway W
P.O. Box 509
Wausau, WI 54402-0509

Ohio River Ginseng
    and Fur, Inc.
P.O. Box 2347
Route 267
East Liverpool, OH 43920

Progenix Corporation
1013 North 3rd Avenue
Suite 8
Wausau, WI 54401

Roots O Gold
Box 92
Le Center, MN 56057

Wilcox Natural Products
P.O. Box 391
161 Howard Street
Boone, NC 28607

SOIL, LEAF, AND SEED ANALYSIS LABORATORY

Dr. Akhtar Khwaja
K Ag Laboratories
    International, Inc.
2323 Jackson Street
Oshkosh, WI 54901

FABRIC SHADE SOURCES

Dave and Katy Lemke
Blacken Lake Shade and Shang
W6869 Cedar Street
Medford, WI 54451

Dayton Bag and Burlap
P.O. Box 8
322 Davis Avenue
Dayton, OH 45401

Gintec Shade Technologies,
    Inc.
RR 1
Windam Center, Ontario
Canada NOE 2AO

Progenix Corporation
1013 North 3rd Avenue
Suite 8
Wausau, WI 54401

Shade Tree Privacy and
    Shade Screen
Yonah Manufacturing
    Company
P.O. Box 1415
Cornelia, GA 30531

Canadians interested in learning more
about ginseng cultivation can contact:

Ginseng Growers Association
    of Canada
395 Queensway West
Simcoe, Ontario
Canada N3Y 2N4

Bibliography

Hardacre, Val. *Woodland Nuggets of Gold.* Northville, MI: Holland House Press, 1974.

Harding, A. R. *Ginseng and Other Medicinal Plants.* Columbus, OH: A. R. Harding Publishing Company, 1908.

Harriman, Sarah. *The Book of Ginseng.* New York: Pyramid Publications, 1976.

Heffern, Richard. *The Complete Book of Ginseng.* Millbrae, CA: Celestial Arts, 1976.

Jartoux, Pierre. *The Description of a Tartarian Plant, called Gin-seng: with an Account of its Virtues.* Paris: 1713 (London: 1714).

Kimmens, Andrew C. *Tales of the Ginseng.* New York: William Morrow & Company, 1975.

Lee, Florence C. *Facts about Ginseng, the Elixer of Life.* Elizabeth, NJ: Hollym International Corp., 1992.

Parke, J. L., and K. M. Shotwell. *Diseases of Cultivated Ginseng.* Publication A3465. Madison, WI: University of Wisconsin-Extension, 1989.

Pritts, Kim D. *American Ginseng: Forest Gold.* Mount Joy, PA: Pritts Enterprises, 1985.

Veninga, Louise. *The Ginseng Book.* Felton, CA: Big Tree Press, 1973.

Washington, George. *Diaries of George Washington,* vol. 4. Donald Jackson and Dorothy Twohig, eds. Charlottesville, VA: University Press of Virginia, 1978.

ABOUT THE AUTHOR

Kim Derek Pritts, a lifelong outdoor enthusiast, has some thirty years' experience growing and hunting ginseng. A graduate of the agricultural sciences program at the Pennsylvania State University, he has written articles on ginseng and other subjects for numerous magazines, including *Field and Stream, Outdoor Life, Sports Afield,* and *Herb Quarterly.* He has done consulting work on ginseng cultivation for the past ten years. Pritts lives in Lancaster County, Pennsylvania, where he serves as a state conservation officer.

Index